FREE FROM THE PAST

By the same author
A Child at Any Cost?

Free from the Past

MARY MEALYEA

KINGSWAY PUBLICATIONS
EASTBOURNE

Biblical quotations are from the
New International Version © International Bible Society
1973, 1978, 1984. Published by Hodder & Stoughton

Front cover photo by Nigel Blythe, Cephas Picture Library

British Library Cataloguing in Publication Data
Mealyea, Mary
    Free from the past.
    1. Medicine. Psychiatry. Christian viewpoints
    I. Title
    261.5

ISBN 0-86065-594-6

Production and printing in Great Britain for
KINGSWAY PUBLICATIONS LTD
1 St Annes Road, Eastbourne, E Sussex BN21 3UN by
Nuprint Ltd, 30b Station Road, Harpenden, Herts AL5 4SE.

To Mark, William and Emily
with all my love.

Acknowledgements

I would like to acknowledge my gratitude to a number of people who have helped me in the writing of this book: to Alison Bird and Rosemary Lincoln who helped me at various stages with typing; to Dr Mary Philip and Dr Tom Brown, two psychiatrist friends, for their careful reading of my manuscript, helpful comments and encouragement; to Dr Monty Barker for kindly writing a foreword; and finally to my husband Harry whose constant love and encouragement have made this book possible.

In order to preserve confidentiality, all the names in the book have been changed.

Contents

Foreword

In recent years there have been many books written for professional counsellors, mostly from a particular and rather limited counselling standpoint. Here however we have a book which will meet the need of ordinary church members. For it is written by someone who is a doctor and has worked in psychiatry; but she has also faced disappointment and crises and taken apparent wrong turnings in her own life. These Dr Mary Mealyea is willing to share with us, and so she writes not only as a doctor but also as a woman, a mother and a minister's wife. There are no miracle answers, but Dr Mealyea gives us some very practical pointers to ways in which we can begin to allow the grace of God to work in us and transform our lives so that we are no longer trapped in our past.

I warmly recommend this book to all those who have experienced the struggle to understand and break free from past difficulties and failures, and to those who have friends and members of their families and church congregations for whom this is true.

Montagu Barker

Dr Barker is a consultant psychiatrist at the Bristol Royal Infirmary and Churchwarden at Christchurch, Clifton.

Preface

In recent years I have been impressed by the number of people I come across who are struggling with their lives mainly because of events which have taken place in their past. In my work as a doctor in psychiatry and now with CARE Trust, and as a minister's wife, I have spent time with people who have shared their problems with me. Often it becomes obvious that the issues surrounding their problems are either complicated by, or wholly caused by, their past experiences of life. It is almost as if they are imprisoned by their past.

We are all affected to some extent by our past. This book is written for those who feel their past hangs heavy around their necks, bowing them low under its weight.

Many Christians groan inwardly and suffer mental anguish because their experience seems to deny the glorious freedom promised by Jesus. The freedom which is promised is wonderfully wide ranging and comprehensive, and yet many Christians feel as if they are struggling helplessly in a straight jacket.

As we proceed in our Christian lives we become aware of the varieties of freedom which become ours in Christ. With great relief we discover the first of these to be freedom from the condemning power of God's law. As we learn more about this freedom and experience it in our lives we are able to sing with increasing joy the great words of Charles Wesley's hymn, 'No condemnation now I dread; Jesus, and all in him, is mine!'

The second freedom to which Christ calls us is freedom from guilt. Guilt is responsible for a great deal of both physical and mental illness. However, this need not be—Jesus offers us freedom. As we experience the reality that Christ's death is the means of enjoying forgiveness for our sins, like Christian in John Bunyan's *Pilgrim's Progress*, we feel a great burden roll from off our shoulders.

A third freedom which we experience is freedom from the power of sin. Paul writes this to the Romans: 'You have been set free from sin and have become slaves to righteousness' (Rom 6:18). We belong to a new master. We no longer need to answer the call of our old one. We have been adopted into God's family and are heirs together with Christ. This does not mean that we no longer sin. 1 John 1:8 makes this clear, 'If we claim to be without sin, we deceive ourselves and the truth is not in us.' But when we sin we have free and unhindered access to the Father, through Jesus, to receive forgiveness and grace to begin again. We are not enslaved to sin nor do we need to live under its power. Yes, we are free from the power of sin, yet many of us live as if we were still under that power.

Jesus has broken off the shackles in these important areas, and that is glorious; but the burden of my concern is that we might grasp one further dimension of the liberty to which Jesus calls us—freedom from the past.

I

Slaves to the Past

If the Son sets you free, you will be free indeed. (Jn 8:36)

Ann was the kind of person you found yourself instinctively trying to avoid. If you were unfortunate enough to be engaged in conversation by her you knew you would not be free for at least an hour. Ann was always full of moans and groans, for life just never seemed to go smoothly for her. There was always some crisis happening, of which you were compelled to hear every detail. Even if there was nothing particular to worry Ann at that moment she would still worry; she was full of 'ifs' and 'buts' and always imagined the worst. She complained endlessly about all those around her who could never understand the wounds unjustly inflicted on her by her circumstances.

If anyone tried gently to reproach Ann for her inability to cope with even the most minor of life's irritations and for her constant worrying, her reply was always the same, 'I'm just a chip off the old block. My mother was exactly like me, *I can't help it.*'

Instead of enjoying our freedom many of us, like Ann, are overwhelmed by a sense of struggling from day to day, at times barely able to keep our heads above water. So engulfed are we by problems that we begin to imagine we are trying unsuccessfully to navigate our lives through a minefield.

'You, my brothers were called to be free' (Gal 5:13). Paul's words seem to mock us. Where is this freedom? We seem to be imprisoned by every crisis we meet, and totally incapacitated by an inability to cope. Why is it? Are we not able to learn to cope? Is something lacking in our personality? Is it our genes? Are we, as Ann argues, 'a chip off the old block'? What about those memories and events in the past which hang around our necks like great millstones, constantly dragging us down?

Although he had been a Christian for several years, Alan never looked happy. When you spoke with him you always sensed a barrier, as if you could never really get through to the real Alan. There was a cynicism about his attitude to life, and a bitterness which his conversion to Christ hadn't seemed to reach.

As you got to know Alan it wasn't long before you discovered the root of these problems, because Alan frequently made mention of it. When he was fourteen years old his mother had walked out on him, his father and younger sister. She had left to go with another man. Alan's world fell apart. He felt rejected and abandoned. He had never been able to forget the memory of those painful subsequent years nor been able to forgive his mother.

This inability to cope with his past effectively incarcerated Alan in a time warp. It prevented him from entering fully into the joy of the Christian life. He couldn't live his life to the full. He was too busy nursing his past wounds and painful memories, almost as if he were carefully keeping them alive, and allowing them to cast a shadow over every present and future event in his life.

Reluctant freemen

On the cross Jesus won for us the title of princes and heirs, yet we live as though we have discarded the prize. We are content to go around in spiritual rags looking more like beggars than the sons and daughters of the living God. God intends us to wear the royal livery of heaven, to be what Thomas Watson the Puritan writer described as the 'blood royal of heaven'.[1] We are to draw on the capital in the royal reserves and to press on to reach spiritual maturity. Being a 'spiritual giant' is not for a select few as so many of us seem to think. We may hide behind excuses which determine for us lives of mediocrity. Are we content to be paupers in experience and dwarfs in grace? God offers us so much more.

The freedom which Jesus offers us is real but we often fail to take hold of it. After the American Civil War all black slaves were granted freedom. However, many chose to remain in slavery. A slave's life was all they had ever known and they were afraid of the unknown. They were happier and felt more secure in their familiar setting. Others, who did accept freedom, still cringed with fear in the presence of their former masters, and were unable fully to enjoy their newfound freedom for fear of imagined repercussions from their previous owners.

We too can be afraid to accept Christ's freedom for fear of what it might mean to our lives.

Most of us react in one of two ways to our inability to cope with life despite all of God's promises of grace to help us do so. First there are those of us who look around wistfully, seeing other Christians who are coping with the pressures of life, and we wonder why we can't.

'Life hasn't treated them as harshly as it has me. If only they had to endure all the hardships I've had to. That would soon wipe that smug Christian smile from their faces. They wouldn't have that air of poise if they had the financial worries I have.' What we are really saying is that our particular problem is too difficult for God.

Or we can't imagine the possibility of being other than we are; so preoccupied are we with our own struggle that we are unaware of any other way of living the Christian life. We may never have even tried to find out what riches in Christ are available to us.

This kind of attitude is beautifully illustrated in C S Lewis's Narnia story *The Last Battle*. Some dwarfs along with the heroes and heroines of the book had been thrown into a stable during a great battle, but instead of finding themselves in the dirty smelly stable they actually stepped into a beautiful land. However, the dwarfs seemed unable to comprehend this; the others could see where they were, but the dwarfs were oblivious to their new surroundings. The others went over to see them;

> Lucy led the way and soon they could all see the Dwarfs. They had a very odd look. They weren't strolling about or enjoying themselves (although the cords with which they had been tied seemed to have vanished) nor were they lying down and having a rest. They were sitting very close together in a little circle facing one another. They never looked round or took notice of the humans till Lucy and Tirian were almost near enough to touch them. Then the Dwarfs all cocked their heads as if they couldn't see any-one but were listening hard and trying to guess by the sound what was happening.

"Look out!" said one of them in a surly voice. "Mind where you're going. Don't walk into our faces!"

"All right!" said Eustace indignantly. "We're not blind. We've got eyes in our heads."

"They must be darn good ones if you can see in here," said the same Dwarf whose name was Diggle.

"In where?" asked Edmund.

"Why you bone-head, in *here* of course," said Diggle. "In this pitch-black, poky, smelly little hole of a stable."

The lion Aslan, who represents Jesus in the book, appeared at this point, and Lucy appealed to him to do something to help the Dwarfs.

"Dearest," said Aslan, "I will show you both what I can, and what I cannot, do."

The story continues.

Aslan raised his head and shook his mane. Instantly a glorious feast appeared on the Dwarfs' knees: pies and tongues and pigeons and trifles and ices, and each Dwarf had a goblet of good wine in his right hand. But it wasn't much use. They began eating and drinking greedily enough, but it was clear that they couldn't taste it properly. They thought they were eating and drinking only the sort of things you might find in a Stable. One said he was trying to eat hay and another said he had got a bit of an old turnip and a third said he'd found a raw cabbage leaf. And they raised golden goblets of rich red wine to their lips and said "Ugh! Fancy drinking dirty water out of a trough that a donkey's been at! Never thought we'd come to this." But very soon every Dwarf began suspecting that every other Dwarf had found something nicer than he had, and they started grabbing and snatching, and went on to quarrelling, till in a few minutes there was a free fight and all the good food was smeared on their faces and clothes or trodden under foot. But when at last they sat down to nurse their black eyes and their bleeding noses, they all said:

17

"Well, at any rate there's no Humbug here. We haven't let anyone take us in. The Dwarfs are for the Dwarfs."

"You see," said Aslan. "They will not let us help them. They have chosen cunning instead of belief. Their prison is only in their own minds, yet they are in that prison."[2]

We cannot press the illustration too far, but are not many of us a bit like the Dwarfs; oblivious of all that Christ has provided for us and in a prison of our own making?

Gillian, a pretty thirty-year-old, could never understand why her friendships didn't last long. Although she was pleasant in appearance, her personality was not so attractive. She constantly seemed to offend people as she believed in speaking her mind. Why couldn't people understand that she didn't mean to offend—it was just her personality? But it was more than that; she herself was easily offended and often took umbrage if she didn't get her own way. I remember speaking to her one day about this aspect of her personality. She was convinced that she could never change. Why couldn't people accept her the way she was? 'Anyway,' she rationalised, 'I've prayed about it and nothing happens.'

Slave of personality

Like Gillian, many of us see our problems rooted in the type of personality we have. Not that we claim to understand our personality; in fact many aspects of it bewilder us. We wonder why we seem to be so easily provoked to anger and rage. Why are we so easily offended, always putting our foot in it and offending others? We may feel inadequate and unable to make decisions, or we may be painfully shy and unable to relate to people around us. On the other hand, our extrovert and insensitive nature may constantly get us into difficult situations, hurting many in the process. We assume that these characteristics are part and parcel of our temperament, over which we have no control. It seems as if we are slaves of our personality. As I pondered these difficult questions I wondered if we might find some of the answers in our past.

For Gillian part of the problem was that she had been completely spoiled as a child. She had wanted for nothing. Her parents were quite wealthy and they doted on their only child. Gillian had never been taught how to handle being denied anything, for her tears had always brought the desired response for her. Her outspoken remarks as a child had been thought funny and quaint by her parents, but now that she was an adult her behaviour was socially unacceptable. Was Gillian then the victim of her past, and is there no hope of her changing?

A hopeless case?

If we are Christians we can ask God to change the offending aspects of our personality, but when our personality is not immediately changed for the better we conclude that God is either unable or unwilling to do anything about it. Our conclusions are wrong. God is neither unable nor unwilling, but it may be that the direction of our prayers is wrong. Rather than asking God to change our personality, perhaps we need to ask God to help us to understand why we behave the way we do. One of the keys to this lies in understanding our past and how it has influenced the development of our personality.

Transparent but whole

God wants us to be transparent Christians, not so full of complexes that no one, least of all ourselves, can understand us. God wants us to be beautiful people through whom his Spirit flows, demonstrating the fruit of his presence in our lives. God wants us to be able to cope with the pressures of life, be they the pressures of our domestic situations, our work situations or the pressures of our past. He doesn't want us to crumble in a heap with each new crisis (though when we do he is always ready to pick us up). God wants us to be whole people, not fragmented by the hang-ups of the past. In Christ we can know freedom.

How do we experience the reality of that freedom in our lives? Understanding how these complexes and problems in our personality have developed and grown can help. So too can understanding a little of how our past imprisons and influences our behaviour.

2

The Past Unmasked

Andrew was a faithful member of his church: he was there every Sunday without fail. He used to collect, in his car, one or two of the older folk who found it difficult to get on and off buses. On his way out of church he always thanked the minister for his message and said how helpful he had found it. The minister and the rest of the congregation were very impressed with Andrew, and everyone thought he was a fine Christian.

What they didn't know was that Andrew had the most furious temper which was easily aroused. Ever since he was a young child, Andrew had had problems controlling his temper. He didn't understand why, but little things which irritated him could make him suddenly fly into a rage. His wife and children bore the brunt of this and had the bruises to prove it. Andrew was too ashamed of his behaviour and bewildered by it to confide in anyone. When the family went to church they put on their Sunday masks and pretended to everyone that they were a happy family.

Removing the masks

Because there may be so much in our past that we are ashamed of, or embarrassed about, we do our best to pretend it isn't there. We like to impress people with our achievements and hide our failures, and we wear masks to hide our true selves. We are afraid that if people see us as we really are or know all about us they won't want to be our friends or even associate with us.

Our Sunday masks are perhaps our most protective. In church we are particularly keen to be well thought of. We may assume the garb of angels and yet throughout the week let it slip or discard it altogether. We seem to have more in common with fallen angels than we care to admit.

Sometimes we have a whole wardrobe full of masks: a different one for each of our different sets of friends and the different situations we find ourselves in. We may even have a mask to put on before we look in the mirror at ourselves.

We may be very successful in fooling others; we may even be tolerably successful at fooling ourselves; but we can never fool God. God sees us as we are. There is no mask which he cannot penetrate, but all too often we are more concerned about what our fellow Christians think of us than about what God thinks. Before we can know the freedom from the past which Jesus offers us, we may need to allow him to remove our masks. God never abandons us as hopeless cases but he does require us to be honest with ourselves and with him.

Had Andrew and his wife been more honest with the folk in their church and their minister, they might have found help and prayerful support to enable Andrew to deal with his quick temper. There is of course a danger in sharing too openly with too many people. We need to guard the privacy of our marriage relationship and not needlessly embarrass our partner or other family members in public. There is a difference between open, caring and honest relationships within our churches and going around sharing all the personal details of our lives with everyone we meet. Sharing and being honest with others has to be done in a prayerful and sensitive manner. It must not be done in order to gain attention, but rather to receive help.

Andrew needed to accept that he had a problem. Wearing a mask over it on a Sunday only made the problem worse. Rather than praying simply that God will change the undesirable aspects of our personality, we need to ask him to tear away the many masks that hide our true selves, and to help us to see ourselves as we really are, recognising what our problems are.

'There is no slavery that can compare to the ingrained habits of sin' (Richard Foster).[1] Andrew had prayed that God would take his hot temper away, but he was constantly disappointed when God did not remove it. Andrew needed rather to ask God to help him to be brave enough to take his mask off and seek help. He needed to understand why he kept losing control. In Andrew's case it was simply that as a child he had learned the habit of behaving aggressively when his will was thwarted, and he needed to unlearn it. It was as simple as that. But Andrew had convinced himself he was ill.

We cannot expect to enjoy the full benefits of our relationship with Christ if we insist on wearing masks. We should not be surprised that we do not know the freedom Christ offers us if we continue to refuse to be honest with ourselves.

Many of us carry around an overloaded filing cabinet on our backs, crowded out with memories and events from the past which weigh us down. Some of these memories have been pushed to the back of our filing cabinet and out of conscious awareness. All we are left with is the effect they have on our personality and therefore on our behaviour.

Have we reached the point where we imagine that God has despaired of us? That God has raised his hands in horror and decided to abandon us as hopeless cases?

After his triple denial of Christ, Peter must have felt himself to be just that, a hopeless case. These events which were now part of Peter's past could have destroyed him. They could have caused him to separate himself from the other disciples and from Jesus—a not uncommon reaction to past sin. However, in John 21 we find Peter with the rest of the disciples eating with Jesus. We can almost imagine Peter slinking in a corner, eager to be near Jesus and yet utterly devastated by and ashamed of his denial of him, wanting to see Jesus and yet frightened of being seen by him. Jesus tenderly, yet firmly, draws Peter out into the open. Even though we frequently let Jesus down he never lets us down. We may even deny him but he will never deny nor abandon us.

We do not need to be afraid of taking off our masks before God or man. Indeed the effort of wearing a mask produces, at times, intolerable strain and stress. We cannot deal with the past by putting a mask over it.

Having honest relationships with God and other people will lead to a healthier mental and physical state.

3

The Great Escape

A fallen world

Inevitably as we grow up we are tainted by the effects
of the fallen world in which we live. We are born in sin
and raised in a sinful world. The harsh realities of life
and the way many lead their lives may leave deep
impressions on us. Some have childhood memories
which they would rather forget, but the effects of them
are not so easy to leave behind. Indeed, we cannot
reach adulthood without being damaged by some
wounds. Some of these wounds are superficial and
leave little trace, while others are deep and cause large
scars.

The environment in which we grow up must inevitably influence our character development. We learn,
often without even realising, patterns of behaviour
from parents, relatives and friends, patterns which can
in later life hinder our spiritual growth as Christians.

New creatures

'Therefore, if anyone is in Christ, he is a new creation;
the old has gone, the new has come!' (2 Cor 5:17) Does
this mean that what happened to us before we became
Christians no longer has any bearing on our lives? Is

our past simply erased? Can we completely abandon it? Certainly our experience would deny this possibility.

'Before I formed you in the womb I knew you, before you were born I set you apart; I appointed you as a prophet to the nations' (Jer 1:5). Jeremiah was left in no doubt that God had been interested in his past. And God is interested in our past too. We cannot simply dismiss it when we become Christians. Sweeping it under the carpet won't do. God's plans for us include our past.

A change of direction

Being 'in Christ' means having changed direction. When we become Christians we leave the path which leads to destruction, to follow that which leads to eternal life. We move out of the realm in which sin rules to enter the kingdom of God where sin has no power over us. We also have a change of masters. We may have been unaware of being the slaves of Satan, but Satan claims all those who do not own Christ as Lord. As Christians we now owe allegiance to Christ, and as such acknowledge his kingship in our lives.

If we have lived careless lives for some period of time, lying, cheating, deceiving, or even just being wrapped up in ourselves, we will not change overnight into sweet, gentle, forebearing and selfless creatures. If we have been shy, introverted people we will not suddenly become gregarious and extrovert. Nor vice versa. If we have struggled all our lives with stress and anxiety, unable to cope with the pressures of life, we will not immediately become the kind of people who tackle problems effortlessly. Personality and psychological problems will not vanish at conversion.

What will change immediately will be the rules by which we lead our lives, the direction of our lives, our aims and desires. As we go on in the Christian life we will discover a growing desire to put Christ first in our lives. Instead of wanting our own way we will want Christ's ways. Instead of being careless of sin we will become intensely sensitive to it and desire to see it evicted from our lives. Gradually there is an increasing awareness that we are not alone in our problems. Instead of having no one to help us cope adequately with life we can know the power of the Holy Spirit in our lives.

The process whereby our lives change to conform to these new desires and awarenesses may be relatively slow. It will certainly be ongoing and will inevitably involve our dealing with and coming to terms with our past.

Martyn Lloyd Jones has written these words: 'The fundamental elements in our personality and temperament are not changed by conversion and rebirth. The new man means the new disposition, the new understanding, the new orientation, but the man himself psychologically is essentially what he was before.'[1]

Does this imply that if we have personality or psychological problems there is nothing that can be done to help us? Surely not. It is my firm belief that there is no one beyond God's help. There is no personality too difficult for God to help. Nor is there any psychological problem which God cannot enable us to handle.

Our past can effectively incarcerate us in a thick-walled prison. The devil's lie is that there is no way out. From the cross Jesus throws a ladder down to us whereby we may escape, but unless we place our feet on the first rung of that ladder we cannot begin to climb out.

There are some factors which can hinder our progress or even prevent us beginning our escape:

Instant success?

One of the first things which may dampen our enthusiasm is our unsatisfied desire for an instant cure. I mentioned in the last chapter that when we are looking to God to help us it may be that the direction of our prayers is wrong. It is also the case that the reason for our apparent failure is often that we have a wrong expectation of *how* God will answer our prayers. Many Christians, like Gillian in a previous chapter, want a 'magic cure'; to be able to go to bed one night, hand God their difficult personality and hurtful past and waken up the next morning to find that they are completely changed and their past is no longer a problem. Of course God could do it, but this sort of solution would not encourage our spiritual growth. When a young child is trying to master new skills, it does not help him if an adult immediately steps in and solves every difficulty for him.

We all learn by doing, and so mature in every aspect of our lives. People who become Christians merely to have all their problems solved will be sadly disappointed.

God may not rescue us *from* our difficulties but he will rescue us *in* them. God will not necessarily remove our problems or immediately change our difficult personality, but he will help us to understand why we have these problems and enable us to discover ways of coping and tackling the issues involved. We need to want

28

that help and have a willingness to change. God's methods of teaching us to cope are gracious and gentle—he never bulldozes us. He waits for an invitation into our lives to help us with our problems. He doesn't break down the door with an axe and rush in ready to do battle in our hearts and lives.

Perseverance

We need to keep on climbing the ladder out of our prison. We mustn't give up when the going gets tough or there is no immediate success. Perseverance is one of the hallmarks of the Christian life and often it is tested early on. There may even be a certain anticlimax or period of testing soon after someone has become a Christian. C S Lewis illustrates this point very well in his book *Screwtape Letters* in which a senior devil instructs a junior devil on the practices of 'the enemy' (God).

> The Enemy allows this disappointment to occur on the threshold of every human endeavour. It occurs when the boy who has been enchanted in the nursery by *Stories from the Odyssey* buckles down to really learning Greek. It begins when lovers have got married and begin the real task of learning to live together. In every department of life it marks the transition from dreaming aspiration to laborious doing.[2]

The devil battles to prevent us becoming Christians, and once we have given our lives to Christ he does not consider the battle finished. The area of battle merely changes. His aim is to make us give up. At each hurdle we encounter he is there whispering discouraging thoughts. 'This kind of life is really too hard. What's the point?' The devil seeks to have us settle in the valley of mediocrity rather than soar to the heights of Christian maturity.

Choices

As we persevere in climbing our ladder, despite no immediate signs that things are improving, we will be faced with many choices to make. If we have the idea that when we give our lives to Jesus he takes over completely and we turn into some kind of robot, we are mistaken. If we imagine that becoming a Christian means that we are no longer responsible for making any decisions or choices, then we should not be surprised if we make little progress as a Christian.

In fact when we become Christians Jesus frees us to make more choices. He enables us, but doesn't force us, to make right choices. The way we think and choose to react in situations will no longer be determined by a fallen nature but by our new nature. We do not need to be trapped by our past patterns of behaviour or emotional reactions; we can make new choices. Nor do we need to be in bondage to the past; we are free in the fullest and truest sense.

In the previous chapter Andrew was faced with a choice—to continue to wear a mask over his unbridled temper or face his true self and seek help to change. Gillian too had to choose: she could remain a slave to her past or choose freedom in Christ. Alan's choices were to allow his past experience with his mother to continue to make him distrust everyone in the present or future, or to put his past behind him, forgive his mother and move out into a fuller and happier life in the present.

A simple enough solution? Even if we are able to see

our situation that clearly, finding the strength to make the choice may seem impossible. We need to ask ourselves how important it is for us to change. The answer to that question will help us know whether success is within our grasp or not. If we see the need to change as vitally important, in fact so important that we are willing to say to God, 'My relationship with you is *the* most important thing in all the world to me, and anything which is hindering that relationship must be dealt with, no matter the cost,' then God will see to it that we do not fail. But it really has to be that important to us. If on the other hand we think it would be nice to change, but perhaps later on, or at least as long as it doesn't upset me or all my plans, then we are almost inevitably doomed to failure.

In other words we need motivation, and for the Christian that motivation springs from a whole-hearted desire to be the very best for God.

Angry jailor

If we are making progress in escaping our past, not expecting a magic cure, persevering in the midst of difficulties and making new choices for our lives, we should not be surprised if the devil is a little unhappy. He wants us to remain in our prison. He doesn't want us to escape because that will mean we will be of more use to God. Indeed, we should expect his counter attacks and sabotage attempts. One of Satan's most successful ways of keeping us imprisoned is to convince us that there is no way out. He cunningly argues, 'The way you are is the way you will always be. You can't change. Jesus gives you salvation and forgiveness but he can't do anything about your personality and temperament—that is already formed and forged from the past. And anyway doesn't Jesus accept you the way you are?' The devil throws in a little bit of truth just to authenticate his lies.

I have frequently heard Christians explain and excuse their short temper and abrasive personality by saying something like this; 'I just call a spade a spade and if Jesus accepts me as I am so can everyone else.'

The amazing thing is that Jesus does accept us the way we are, warts and all. But that doesn't mean that he is pleased with our behaviour or that he doesn't intend us to change. We grieve him by our refusal to allow the Spirit of God to work in our lives and enable us to change and be transformed into the likeness of Christ.

> Therefore, I urge you, brothers, in view of God's mercy, to offer your bodies as living sacrifices, holy and pleasing to God—this is your spiritual act of worship. Do not conform any longer to the pattern of this world, but be transformed by the renewing of your mind. Then you will be able to test and approve what God's will is—his good, pleasing and perfect will (Rom 12:1–2).

Low expectations

Another ploy of the devil is to encourage us to have low expectations of the Christian life. We are satisfied if we don't commit any 'big sins', if we remain relatively chaste and attend church reasonably regularly. We convince ourselves that the 'deeper life' is for others. 'It is too high for the likes of us. We can't all be an Amy Carmichael or a Hudson Taylor. It's all right if we sin a little bit, now and again.'

A W Tozer in *Leaning into the Wind* has this to say about such thinking; 'The "deeper life" is deeper only because the average Christian life is tragically shallow.'[3]

How do we change?

There is no denying that many Christians have genuine problems in their personality or psychological make-up. These make it extremely difficult for them to cope with the pressures of life. Life is more of an endurance test than a pleasure. They may have tried very hard to overcome their problems without success and are discouraged. Others feel trapped by the circumstances they find themselves in and are unable to escape from their environment. This is especially true where the problem is within the marriage or family.

How do we cope? Is it possible to become the kind of people who can handle problems whatever they be? Before we can face the present we need to deal adequately with the past. Many of us are so busy coping with our past lives and problems that we are unable fully to enjoy the present. So intent are we to nurse old wounds and scars that we are not free to give our full attention to present affairs. Nor are we free to allow our personalities to change and grow. We may be unconscious of doing this and may even fiercely deny it.

None of us is immune from the pressures the world applies to us. From the moment we are born these pressures begin and not even as Christians do we escape. We are not born wearing protective clothing to shield us against the harmful influences around us. The deep scars inflicted on us may prevent our full enjoyment of Christ as he intends. But it doesn't need to remain like this.

There are Christians who come to Christ for salvation weighed down by a burden of guilt. This burden is eased by conversion and the knowledge of forgiveness. But they still allow the memories to haunt them.

There are others who have been so badly treated in childhood that they have lost the ability to trust anyone. They even have difficulty trusting God.

Others still have had no experience of loving relationships and therefore find it difficult in later life to make friends or relate to people on any level.

The devil can use our past memories and scars to imprison us, convincing us that our ingrained patterns of behaviour and temperament are a permanent part of us. We can use this as an excuse to abrogate all responsibility for the way we behave.

But there is healing for the scars life inflicts on us. We can unlearn maladaptive behaviour patterns. Jesus has thrown a ladder of escape—a lifeline—into our prison. He can free us from the negative influences of our past and help us to become whole people. God created man in his own image. Sin has marred that image. Jesus came to restore it. Will we let him restore it fully? Will we take that first step onto the ladder of escape?

'Now to him who is able to do immeasurably more than all we ask or imagine, according to his power that is at work within us, to him be glory in the church and in Christ Jesus throughout all generations, for ever and ever! Amen' (Eph 3:20–21).

4

The Past in the Present

Rejection

I met Catherine several years ago. She had been a
Christian for some time and was now in her mid-
thirties. Superficially she seemed to be getting on fine in
her Christian life: she had served God in a variety of
ways over the years. My first contact with her was
through a mutual friend. For some time Catherine had
been experiencing increasing tension until she could no
longer face speaking to anyone.

As her story unfolded I became aware of a great deal
of unhappiness in Catherine's early life. She had never
been able to please or satisfy her overbearing parents.
Her father was very strict with her and frequently
resorted to physical punishment right up to her late
teen years. When Catherine tried to please her mother
by helping around the house her mother would respond
with criticism and re-do whatever Catherine had done.

Catherine was never able to satisfy the demands of
her parents and therefore never earned their praise, a
thing which she desperately wanted and needed. There
was little love in the home and Catherine felt herself to
be totally rejected.

Unfortunately her marriage was not a happy one.

Catapulted into it, to escape her unhappy home situation, she married literally the first man who asked her.

This story is not as uncommon as many would think. If Catherine had made a more appropriate choice of marriage partner much of the early harm in her life might have been healed. But as it was her husband was uncannily like her father: overbearing, strict, and seldom gave praise. This served to stir up the awful memories of the past from which there seemed no escape.

Striving for approval

Catherine found herself constantly striving for approval. She worked her fingers to the bone trying to please everyone, looking for the praise and approval she had always longed for and yet was denied as a child and then in her marriage. Most people thought Catherine was a wonderful person; always doing things for people, running after her family, always eager to help—in fact, if truth be told, too eager; often people's initial delight at being helped turned into irritation.

Over the years all this striving had taken its toll on Catherine. The need for approval proved to be a terrible tyrant. Catherine didn't realise she was striving for approval; all she was aware of was her terrible tension and anxiety. When I first suggested to her that this was what she was doing she was surprised, but then it all made sense to her. Until she was able to see what was making her tense and anxious she could never be free from these feelings.

Violated and betrayed

Linda was in her late twenties when I first met her. She always seemed angry and aggressive, and totally unable to relate to people. When she became a Christian she realised that her anger and aggression were wrong, but she was unable to do anything about it. It was so bad that most people learned to steer clear of her in case she bit their heads off.

As I became acquainted with her she shared some of her early experiences of life with me. From a very early age her father had regularly sexually assaulted her. Her mother had an idea of what was going on but never tried to stop it. It wasn't difficult to understand why Linda was always so angry. The real objects of her anger were her father for violating her trust in him and her mother for being a silent partner in the crime. Her mother was now dead, and she didn't know or care where her father was, so she was unable to vent her anger on them. It was easier to project her anger onto everyone else around her.

But the anger inside her, which was never appeased, was strangling her enjoyment of life. Her anger affected not only her relationship with her fellow Christians but also her relationship with God. She found it difficult to believe that he really loved her. Inwardly she was angry with God, for she blamed him for allowing her to endure such a traumatic childhood.

'Anger is an acid which can do more harm to the vessel in which it is stored than to anything on which it is poured' (Anonymous).

Personality

It is not too difficult to see how the past has affected both Catherine's and Linda's personalities. But what exactly do we mean when we speak of personality? Our personality is what makes us unique. *The Oxford Illustrated Dictionary* (Second edition, published by Oxford University Press 1976) describes personality as 'distinctive personal character, and character as 'sum of distinguishing features of an individual'.

Our personality is what separates us from other family members and makes us different from them; the aspects of our nature which stand out or are predominant. What were the special features which stood out about Catherine? She was tense, anxious, and insecure. Similarly Linda was angry and aggressive. The problem areas in our personality are not always so easily identified.

There are several broad categories we can use to classify personality. We will deal only with some of the more familiar ones. The hysterical personality is one which we have all met, the person who craves love and attention yet fears the intimacy of real relationships. Another familiar one is the extrovert, the life and soul of every party. Extreme extroverts seem never to have serious thoughts in their heads. At the other end of the scale is the introvert, the painfully shy person who is always analysing his thoughts and deeds. Of course we also have the Catherines and Lindas of the world and many more. There are many different words we can use to describe someone's personality and these words may convey different meanings to us all, so it can be unwise to label people as one thing or another.

Most reasonably well-adjusted people can display

many of the qualities which we use to categorise people. We are all a bit hysterical from time to time. We can all display histrionic behaviour when it suits us. We may be extrovert at times and introvert at other times. In other words, our personality includes many features and in the well person these are kept in balance. Usually one particular feature is more dominant but we can only speak of someone having a personality disorder or problem when the quality of that person's life, or the life of those around him, is adversely affected.

Although we are unique as individuals the paradox is that the distinctive qualities of our personality will have been shared by countless others. There is no new personality, for human nature remains the same, only the manifestations of it change.

What forms our personality?

For many years now psychologists and others have argued about what forms our personality. Are we merely born introvert and shy or did we learn this type of behaviour from someone else? Or did circumstances contrive to make it inevitable that we would turn out the way we are?

What of those who say our personality is all inherited? We are bad-tempered individuals because we inherited this from a bad-tempered parent and there is nothing that can be done about it. Can we inherit personality traits like quick temper, anxiety, histrionic behaviour, an inability to cope with stress, etc?

Genetic code

At the moment of conception we inherit what is known as a genetic code. This determines how we develop in the uterus. First of all it determines that we develop into human beings rather than cats or dogs. It also determines things like hair colour, skin colour, eye colour and our general body shape and size. There are several diseases we may inherit. And to *some* extent we inherit our intellectual capacity and emotional temperament. We may inherit a general disposition or tendency towards being happy and outgoing. Or we may inherit a tendency to be strong willed and rebellious of authority. We may inherit a degree of difficulty in coping with stress. However, this does not mean that these tendencies will automatically be firm features of our personality.

Environment

From the moment of conception another factor impinges upon and influences our genetic code, and that factor is our environment. From the time we are conceived there is a constant interaction between our environment and our genetic code which determines how we develop and this goes on for the whole of our lives.

We are born with the genetic material which allows us to learn to speak. If our mother develops rubella (German Measles) while we are developing in her uterus, we may be born with the congenital abnormality of deafness. (Congenital means existing before or at the time of birth.) Therefore although we have the ability, genetically, to learn to speak, we will not do so

40

because we cannot hear sounds and words to copy. Another special environment will have to be created before we can learn to speak.

We may be born to parents who are both brilliant in the academic world and inherit the best possible genes for intellectual development. However, if brain injury occurs at birth we will be mentally retarded.

So too with our personality. We may inherit a general tendency towards a particular type of temperament. However, our environment begins to affect it from the moment we are born. Every parent knows that a child has definite likes and dislikes from the moment it is born. Where there is more than one child in the family, parents will testify readily that each child has demonstrated different characteristics from a very early stage. Some babies are born with what seems to be a constant cheerful disposition—easily contented and pacified. Others come into the world determined to rule everyone in sight and be pleased by nothing.

As children we are totally dependent on those caring for us to determine our environment. We may be fortunate and have a happy environment in which to grow up, or we can become the victims of uncaring, insensitive or even cruel parents and circumstances. A naturally happy and content child can quickly turn into an unhappy one if it is starved of love and attention. A child who has a strong will and stubborn nature can turn into a delinquent if not handled correctly. However, the same child, given the right environment and set of parents, may turn into a world leader.

Our genetic pattern is determined at conception when we receive half our genetic code from our father and the other half from our mother. There is nothing we can do to alter this after conception (barring genetic engineering). On the other hand our environment, which is constantly changing and influencing us, can be changed and its effect on us modified.

It is obvious to see how circumstances shaped Catherine's personality. But wait a minute—we could argue that her sister, who grew up in the same environment, turned out all right. Perhaps she would have had a nervous disposition no matter what her childhood had been like. Perhaps that's the way she was born and she irritated her parents with her behaviour so that it was her effect on them which made them react to her in the way they did.

What about Linda? Surely it is more obvious that the trauma of her childhood affected her to make her angry and aggressive. But her father was an angry and aggressive man. Perhaps she really inherited it from him—or maybe she learned it from him?

The arguments about heredity versus environment will no doubt go on for a long time yet. But the question, 'Is our personality due to our genes or our environment?' is too simplistic. The answer must embrace a combination of both.

Modelling

By the time we reach adulthood there will have been many factors working on our personality. Besides our environment and genetic make-up there is also a process called 'modelling' going on.

Jack grew up in a family where his father was very aggressive and rude towards his wife (Jack's mother). Jack never saw his parents showing each other affection. They constantly quarrelled, and often Jack's dad hit his mum. Jack's father took his wife for granted and

Jack's mother showed nothing but contempt for her husband. She reacted to all this by retreating to her bed complaining of a headache and feeling sick.

Children model themselves on the adults closest to them. Little boys tend to use their dad as their model and little girls model themselves on their mums, although they learn from both parents and indeed from all other adults with whom they have a close relationship.

What kind of example had Jack been given on which to model his own behaviour? He learned to treat women harshly. He learned to react in situations by becoming angry and aggressive. He didn't learn much about affection or caring for people. What did he learn from his mother? He saw her walking away from the situation. She didn't face up to her problems. She reacted by developing neurotic symptoms.

A couple whom I knew spent most of their time arguing with each other. They once said to me that they were puzzled about why their children were always arguing with each other and couldn't get on together. I asked them if they felt that the fact that they didn't get on well and were always fighting had anything to do with it. They seemed surprised by my question.

Another friend once complained to me that her little girl of ten was always telling lies. I asked her if she ever told lies. At first she denied this and then later admitted that she only told 'white lies' which surely didn't count. As parents we may believe our behaviour is quite innocent. For example, someone telephones to speak to your husband. You know that he doesn't want to speak to this person so although he is at home you tell the person your husband is out. All of this is done in the presence of your child.

It is not so much that your child learns to lie—that seems to come naturally to us all. Our fallen nature is all too evident in even the youngest of our children. What happens is that the child learns that it is all right to tell lies. Mum and Dad do it. They quickly learn that telling lies is quite acceptable as long as you can justify it. Lying is permissible if it gets you out of trouble or an awkward situation. The habit forms, and then the reason for lying is obscured and becomes irrelevant.

Shaping our lives

It is clearly apparent that our personality and the way we behave greatly affects the way we live our lives. There is nothing we can do about our genetic make up but perhaps, as we have seen, our genes are not as important as many think. Is there anything we can do about the effects of our environment on our personality? Or by the time we reach adulthood is our personality set in concrete? As we look back over our past we begin to see just how important it has been in shaping our personality for good or ill.

5

The Impotent Tyrant

As we saw in the last chapter the environment in which we grow up has a tremendous influence on the development of our personality. In other words, our past influences what we are in the present. However, our 'past' is not confined to our early years, nor is it confined to the environment our parents or guardians determine for us. Undoubtedly these early years, while we are so vulnerable, are extremely important. The influences brought to bear on us during this time are no doubt crucial and formative. But the past does not end once we have outgrown nappies and school uniforms.

Our past goes on right up to a minute ago. Everything that has happened to us in our lives right up to the present can have a profound bearing on what we are, how we behave, and how we respond and react to people and situations.

Skeletons in the cupboard

Most of us have skeletons in our cupboards, old bones which can spring to life with amazing alacrity. Events which we may have considered dead and buried can rise

45

to haunt us. Even things which we feel we have dealt with and put aside can affect our present-day reactions.

The devil takes full advantage of our Achilles' heel and makes sure that our old bones do a great deal of rattling. The noise of their rattling can fill our hearts with fear and forboding.

Rebuke from the past

A chance meeting with an acquaintance or friend from the past can stir unwelcome memories. I was out shopping one day with my friend Jenny when someone stopped to say hello. Gordon spoke to Jenny for just a few seconds, enquiring how she was getting on. Immediately Jenny's colour drained and she became obviously uneasy and tense. It took Jenny forty minutes to recover her composure after that brief encounter, and it spoiled our whole afternoon.

Apparently the friendly hello had sounded to Jenny like a rebuke from the past. It had come from a member of a church that Jenny had belonged to two years previously. The church had been run on strict disciplinary and legalistic lines. Jenny attended it for three years and during that time it had put her in a spiritual straitjacket. It had taken courage finally to decide to leave, and when she did she felt as though she had been liberated from a concentration camp. There had been quite a bit of bad feeling at the time from other folk in the church, who assumed that her leaving meant that she was backsliding. She had in fact joined a very lively evangelical church where the Lord was obviously blessing her.

The acquaintance who said hello to Jenny held no power over her, nor did the church that she had left.

But the unexpected meeting had filled her with a sudden panic. In the early months after her departure, Jenny had purposely tried to avoid anybody from her previous church. This had made her edgy and unable fully to enjoy her new freedom in her new church environment. Even now, two years on, this meeting had the power to stir memories which upset her.

The past can shackle us

If we are honest, most of us would have to admit to some things in our past which we are now either ashamed of or embarrassed about. Some may, like Jenny, have moved on to a new situation and begun to make new friends, but still live in a certain amount of apprehension (if not fear) of the new friends finding out too much about our past. This can effectively shackle us and make us wary of getting too close to people. In this way our past interferes with present day relationships.

In our previous chapter we saw how Linda's anger held her prisoner and prevented her from trusting people and stopped her making friends. I'm sure if we were all to think about our own past we would be able to see how some of our reactions today are governed by events in our past.

Of course, not all events affect us adversely. In my first year at university I didn't apply myself to my work as I should. As a result I failed an exam and had to re-sit it. The experience of having to study all through the summer vacation, and the fear of getting thrown out of medical school if I didn't pass the re-sit was so dreadful that I decided I would make sure I had no more re-sits. That fear helped to prod me into working harder throughout the rest of my medical course. However, if the fear had been greater it could have so paralysed me that I would have been unable to do any work.

Our memories can hold terror and unhappiness which we feel we have successfully filed in the past— until something happens in the present to stir those memories. The devil does his best to see that this happens. If successful in this activity the devil can render us useless or near to it in God's service. We may be unaware of the effect our past is having on us, and we may not be able to experience healing until we are aware of the damage being done to us.

Carol's father was an alcoholic. She couldn't remember a time when life wasn't overshadowed by her father's drinking. Surprisingly Carol's dad had been able to retain his responsible job. But the whole family tried to hide the fact of his drinking, although probably more people knew about it than they realised.

Carol was ashamed of her father and her home situation. As a result she never invited friends home in case they should encounter her drunken father. As she knew she couldn't return invitations to other friend's houses she declined them. This all resulted in Carol becoming shy and unwilling to make friends.

When she became a Christian her shyness and difficulty in making friends became a real handicap to her Christian development. It took her a long time to get to know people in church: she was too frightened they would find out about her dad. So she didn't fully enter into the life of the church or enjoy the benefits of doing so. Her fellowship was threatened and so too was her ability to witness to others about Christ. Everything about her life seemed tinged by the secret she carried around. A dark cloud hung over every friendship and people just wrote her off as being unfriendly.

It was only in later years when she determined to escape her shy personality that she realised that her personality problems were closely related to her past. As she prayed for God to help her she was able to see how her shyness was closely linked to her shame about her father. With God's help she was able to deal with the shame and conquer her shyness. However, it was hard work. Every time she went to church or a Christian gathering she would pray, 'Lord help me to be natural, help me to speak to just one person, help me to be sensitive to the stranger who may be just as terrified of speaking to people as I am.'

It didn't come easily to Carol. Years of being afraid to speak to people had woven itself into a fairly fixed part of Carol's personality. However, she persevered in the face of discouragements. She refused to listen to the lies of the devil who told her that she would never change. Then there came a day when she looked back and realised that the change had taken place. She was no longer afraid of people or of her past. No longer was she eager to sit at the back of the church hoping no one would notice her. No longer did she creep into a crowded room and seek oblivion in some corner of it.

Miracle of exchange

God does not intend us to be prisoners of our past. When we come to Christ and bring him our lives we bring him our past too. We lay our lives in their entirety at the foot of the cross. Then a miracle of exchange takes place. We are united to Christ. Romans 6:5 tells us that our old self is crucified with Christ. In our union with Christ our past becomes his past and his ours. Jesus frees us not only from our own sin but from the sin which has been committed against us. Our past no longer holds any power over us—we have a new past, Christ's past. We are free.

These are the facts of the gospel but our experience is so often quite contrary to this. Our past seems to hold a great deal of power over us.

I remember going to the zoo once and seeing a large ape securely behind bars. All of a sudden the ape threw itself at the bars of its cage and at the same time let out a loud roar. All the onlookers, including myself, jumped back from the cage and gasped in fear. The ape could not harm us but for a moment its lunge at us and its roar made us believe that it could.

So too with our past. Our skeletons are only old bones. They cannot harm us but the noise of their rattling can make us believe that they can. This is what the devil wants us to believe.

No longer has sin any power over us as Christians. We have moved out of that realm where sin has dominion and into God's kingdom where sin has no power. So too the past has no power over us. But the past can still roar at us and sometimes Christians mistake this roaring for power.

6

I Will Remember Your Sins No More

Susan had been a Christian for many years. She had been involved in Christian Union activities while at university and went on to be an active member of an evangelical church. Susan was well respected as a Christian and looked up to by the younger Christians in her circle of friends, but she was desperately lonely. She would go along to church activities with a smile on her face, her mask of happiness, but in her heart she dreaded returning to an empty flat. All her close university friends were married now. Most even had children, and Susan wondered why God had denied her the joy of a marriage partner.

For much of the time Susan was happy and content. For most of the time she was able freely to acknowledge that God's perfect will for her at the moment was singleness. There were many struggles and battles with loneliness which Susan successfully conquered. However there were times when she sank low in the depths of despair, struggling unsuccessfully with her fierce emotions and desire for a partner in life.

It was at precisely one of these low points in Susan's life that she became prey to the attention of a married man in her office. At first she resisted his romantic overtures although aware of a certain attraction to him. She felt flattered and it was a boost for her deflated ego. One day in a particularly vulnerable moment—she had that morning received a wedding invitation from the last of her unattached friends—she accepted an invitation from John to join him for a coffee after work.

Almost immediately after Susan had accepted John's invitation warning bells rang loudly inside her. 'He's a married man—goodness, Susan, what do you think you're doing? This is dangerous. John is far too handsome and charming and you know quite well his intentions are not strictly business.'

And so she struggled with her conscience. She was almost on the point of telephoning through to his office to cancel the arrangement when she finally squashed her conscience. 'I'm a mature Christian, I can handle this situation. I won't let it get out of hand. Anyway, perhaps I can witness to him about my faith. I'm not doing anything wrong—having coffee with a workmate is quite innocent, nobody could criticise. It will be an opportunity to discuss some recent problems at work,' she argued with herself.

It had been a long time since Susan had felt the admiration of someone of the opposite sex and she was quite intoxicated by it. Christian men were too afraid of getting involved to have casual dates. They seemed to imagine you had to be ready with a wedding ring before you even asked a girl out for coffee. Susan knew that she should not give John any false encouragement, but she was almost spellbound by his charm. Time passed quickly. They seemed to have many things in common. They laughed and talked for an hour or more. John showed genuine interest in her. He was sensitive and understanding. She had misjudged him. He was really quite lonely and seemed to have a terrible wife. John had listened to what she had to say as if what she was saying really mattered and was quite important.

Susan went home that night confused but happier than she had been for some time. She had enjoyed John's company very much. Again the warning bells rang. She knew she was playing a dangerous game but brushed the warning aside. She would cope. She wouldn't allow herself to get drawn into anything which was wrong. She had the situation well under control.

Over the next few days Susan found herself thinking more and more about John. She rehearsed over and over in her mind their conversation together. She found herself wishing for another opportunity to spend time with him, and it wasn't long before she had her wish granted. There were many opportunities to meet with John. She convinced herself it was all innocent, but she didn't allow herself to question whether John's wife would agree with that.

The inevitable happened; Susan and John became emotionally involved. What had started out with the appearance of innocence quickly became an entangled web of sin and deceit.

Susan knew in her heart what she was doing was wrong. This wasn't at all like her dreams for a life partner. But John seemed so right for her. They seemed meant for one another. Oh, yes, John wasn't a Christian but he was interested in finding out about her faith. He never tried to stop her going to church and said he never would. Susan was sure he would eventually became a Christian. Perhaps this was God's plan that she should bring him to faith. Of course he was married, but John said it had all been a mistake, he should never have married his wife. Surely God couldn't mean him to stay with someone he didn't love. Eventually Susan convinced herself that she was actually following God's perfect plan for her life. Friends tried to counsel her but she was deaf to their words and blind to her sin.

'But it *feels* right,' she would say. 'I've prayed about it and I'm sure God understands how we both feel. It can't be wrong, we love each other.'

I wish the above account was fiction but alas, not only is it true, but it is also far from being a rare event. When I heard Susan's story my heart went out to her. I could understand her loneliness and deep desire for a husband, a quite legitimate desire. I have many other friends who are single and feel the pain of that intensely. It is not easy to be a single Christian in our modern culture which not only advocates that you have a partner but that you have many partners to satisfy your emotional needs. You stand out as being quite odd if you have no partner of the opposite sex.

Susan was vulnerable. Perhaps Christian friends should have realised this and supported her more. However the fact remains that Susan courted temptation. She knew she was on dangerous ground. She had already resisted John's previous invitations, then she allowed herself to be drawn into further dangerous situations until she was trapped. When we play with our emotions it is like skating on very thin ice. We know we are in danger but we convince ourselves that we will be able to stay on the thicker ice where we are safe. Or more perilously we say to ourselves, 'I'll just sin a little bit and then stop—I really need this little bit of sin but I won't let it go too far and then I'll ask God's forgiveness.' We are only fooling ourselves, because sooner or later we will find ourselves helpless. Sin is an inevitable downward track and the farther along it you go the steeper and faster the descent becomes.

Even at that stage Susan could have escaped, for she had friends who wanted to help. They were prepared to get alongside her and pull her out. But Susan closed her ears quite deliberately and chose rather to listen to the lies of the devil—'it feels right so it must be right'. Few of us can afford to be judgemental of Susan. Who of us has never refused to listen to godly counsel and instead preferred the lies of Satan?

Let's examine Susan's situation in greater detail. It is the way in which this past event is going to affect Susan's future that we are particularly concerned with.

First of all Susan alienated herself from her friends and from her church. She could not bear to hear any criticism of her actions and felt herself to have been thoroughly misunderstood and let down, so she avoided her friends and stopped going to church.

She entrenched herself so deeply in the view that what she was doing was being blessed by God and was part of his plan for her life, that she refused to consider any alternative course of action. In fact she almost had a crusade-like zeal to continue her chosen path.

So convinced was Susan that John's marriage had been a dreadful mistake which must be undone, that she became resentful and angry with John's wife for thinking she had any claims on John whatsoever. She was jealous of John spending any time at all with his wife.

Susan stopped reading her Bible—it held too many challenges to her present attitudes and beliefs. She had to hold on to the belief that she was not sinning. God was allowing all this to happen because he had really intended John for her, so she argued with herself. Their meeting must have been 'meant' she told herself.

She was far from happy but was fully persuaded that once John's divorce was through and they were married all would be well. How foolish the devil makes us, for if we belong to Christ, God will not allow us to be happy in our sin—or at least not for long.

The chance to return

In fact the amazing thing is that despite our sin and disobedience, no matter how wilful it is, God still loves us and longs for our return—just like the prodigal son whose father ran out to meet him with open arms when the sinful and disobedient son returned penitent to him.

Susan's story is not so very different from David and Bathsheba's of three thousand years ago. David too, courted temptation when he was also in a vulnerable emotional state, lonely because his men were off fighting. He was looking for companionship and comfort. I don't believe that when he invited Bathsheba to visit him he even dreamed it would lead to murder. David tried to justify his actions to himself and would not listen to godly counsel. But again the amazing fact is that God loved David far too much to leave him in his sin and here we have the whole point of this chapter. God pursued David by means of his faithful servant Nathan, and even though David truly repented when confronted with the truth of his actions, he still had to live with the consequences. David was fully forgiven and restored to his relationship with God, but he lost the son of his adulterous relationship.

It was several years before Susan responded to God's attempts to restore her. During that time she had become quite bitter. John never did became a Christian as Susan hoped he would. Intermittently she had

attended a local church—really just for appearances,
for her heart was cold and unresponsive to God's word.
She had long since stopped trying to justify her actions;
there was no one to listen.

God graciously drew Susan back to himself and
restored her relationship with him, but Susan had to
live with the consequences of her sin. She was now
unhappily married to a man who cared very little for
God. Susan was full of guilt and remorse, and although
she knew God had forgiven her she found it almost
impossible to forgive herself.

Accepting forgiveness

A much-used and helpful illustration of this is the story
of the piece of wood into which a nail is hammered.
When the nail is removed the hole that it made is still
there. Just as when we hammer sin into our lives it
leaves its mark even after its removal. I believe God
can cover that mark with his love. The mark is still
there but it is full of God's love.

I remember when I first read the story of David and
Bathsheba as an adult I was horrified at what David had
done. I could not believe that a servant of God could
behave in such a way—I am not so naive now. One of the
things which particularly disturbed me was the section
when David was distressed for his dying child.

In 2 Samuel 12 we read of the prophet Nathan's
confrontation with David over his sin with Bathsheba.
David had committed adultery with her and then tried
to cover up his sin. When he was unable to do this he
had Uriah, Bathsheba's husband, killed in battle,
adding murder to his adultery. Then again in order to
make everything *look* all right he married Bathsheba

before the birth of the child by their adulterous union.
When the child eventually died David's distress seemed
to vanish immediately. Like his servants I too was a
little annoyed and perplexed. How could he forget his
sin so soon? However, those who sin and are restored
following repentance would do well to pay attention to
David's word: 'While the child was still alive, I fasted
and wept. I thought, "Who knows? The Lord may be
gracious to me and let the child live." But now that he
is dead, why should I fast? Can I bring him back again?
I will go to him, but he will not return to me' (2 Sam
12:22–23). Then David got on with his life.

Often when, as Christians, we sin and then repent
and enjoy God's gracious forgiveness, we are haunted
for the rest of our lives (or a good part of it) by the
memory of our sin. We are like a crazy man with a dog
which dies. We bury the dead dog with great ceremony
but every now and again we return to the graveside and
dig the dog up! We look at the dog and examine it to
see if it is really dead. We cry over it and then we put it
back in the grave until the next time. This story seems
absurd, but many of us behave exactly like that with
our past sins.

There is a place for remembering past sins. Indeed,
David never did forget his sin; nor did the apostle Paul
ever forget that he had been responsible for the deaths
of many Christians before he himself became a Christian. Our past sin should make us more careful in the
future not to repeat it. We should learn from our past
experience but we must reckon our sin to be dead, just
as we do when we first become Christians. Too many
Christians are hindered by past sin which they have
repented. It has been forgiven, but they keep digging it
up and examining it and grieving for it. There is a place

for leaving it in its grave and getting on with our lives. We will serve God better if we do.

Although David lived with certain consequences of his actions, God still described him in very tender terms, and there is no doubt that David went on to serve God as a faithful servant.

Unless Susan is able to deal with the memories of her sin and accept her forgiven and restored state, her usefulness to God will be severely limited. The devil wants us to be like the man with the buried dead dog. He wants us to keep digging it up again to see if it is really dead and in the process relive the agony of guilt and despair. But in doing this we are really calling God a liar. David took God at his word, and when God told him he was forgiven he believed it. Some of David's most beautiful and helpful psalms were written in response to his belief in God's mercy and forgiveness:

As far as the east is from the west,
so far has he removed our transgressions from us.
As a father has compassion on his children,
so the Lord has compassion on those who fear him;
for he knows how we are formed,
he remembers that we are dust (Ps 103:12–14).

Past sin can become an excuse to take the Christian life easy. We disqualify ourselves from office in the church or Christian service. We feel that the rest of our lives should be spent in crying over and repenting for our past sin. This is not so. This is the lie of the devil because it renders us useless in God's service. God restores us fully as his sons and daughters. God can even use our past sin to make us better servants, although that argument can never be used to excuse sin. In a later chapter we will deal more fully with how God can even use our past sin in his service.

7

Lead Us Not Into Temptation

There are many who think they can treat sin lightly. As long as no one finds out it doesn't really matter what we do! That kind of thinking betrays whose approval we are really concerned to earn, for if it were God's approval which was important to us we would not entertain that kind of thinking. God is all seeing and all knowing; we cannot hide from him. When we sin we offend God. No matter what our sin, it is a sin against God.

When Moses spoke to the Reubenites and Gadites in Numbers 32:23 regarding their promise to help the other Children of Israel take possession of their land, he said to them: 'But if you fail to do this, you will be sinning against the Lord; and you may be sure that your sin will find you out.'

We cannot sin in a vacuum, for when we sin other people are almost inevitably affected. We may think that no one knows about it, but even if our sin is a secret from other people, it can never be from God. One day, either in our present life or in the life hereafter, God will expose it.

The words in Psalm 139:1–4 are for our comfort and encouragement, but they are also a warning, for they remind us that we cannot hide from God. Of course as Christians we should not want to hide from him: our lives should be open and transparent.

> O Lord, you have searched me
> and you know me.
> You know when I sit and when I rise;
> you perceive my thoughts from afar.
> You discern my going out and my lying down;
> you are familiar with all my ways.
> Before a word is on my tongue
> you know it completely, O Lord.

Far-reaching effects

I find it quite frightening to see how the course of our whole lives can be changed in an instant for a moment's gratification of pleasure. A moment's yielding to temptation can create havoc in our lives. When we repent of our sin God is gracious in forgiving us, but we may have to live the rest of our life with the consequences of that sin.

Mary was eighteen. She had recently finished her A Levels at school and was looking forward to going on to university. She had much to look forward to. She was clever and pretty, and was heading for the successful career in law which she was planning. Mary had a boyfriend called Bill and they hoped to get married one day, but they were both young and wanted to finish their education first.

Their friendship started innocently enough. They were good friends and enjoyed each other's company. They shared similar interests in sport and outdoor activities. They both came from Christian backgrounds and had attended many Christian rallies and conferences. At these, there were often seminars on court-ship and the Bible's teaching on the dangers of petting and the sinfulness of premarital sex.

At first holding hands and kissing seemed to satisfy Mary's and Bill's emotional needs. Knowing that they had a long time to wait before their marriage they knew that they should go slowly on the physical side. Occasionally they found it impossible to restrain themselves when they found themselves alone together. They knew that because of this they should guard against being alone too often. However, appetites had been whetted. Individually they both suffered pangs of guilt as they thought of what their parents would think if they knew just how far they were going. Sitting in church they were glad that those around them knew nothing of their secret sin. They seemed oblivious to the fact that God knew.

One night while alone in Mary's house passions ran high. Neither wanted to say no to the other. The experience was too exhilarating to end it. Next month a pregnancy test confirmed Mary's growing fear.

The incident had only lasted a few minutes but now Mary was faced with a terrible dilemma. Her parents wanted her to have an abortion. They were frightened of how this would tarnish their Christian image if it became public. An abortion seemed the sensible way out and could be done quickly and secretly. Mary's parents justified their advice by saying that this was best for Mary as otherwise she wouldn't be able to go to university. Bill wanted to marry her. They were both Christians and knew that an abortion was wrong; but what about both their university courses and their future?

Mary had a terrible row with Bill about it all and

opted for an abortion. A year later she became ill with a depressive illness. She had never got over grieving for the baby she had aborted and was full of guilt and remorse. She ended up failing her university course.

Several years later Mary met and married another man, but didn't tell him about her abortion. He too was a Christian and she was worried that he wouldn't approve and she would lose him. Mary continued to have bouts of depression and her marriage ran into difficulties. Because of her past sexual experience having gone so wrong, Mary found herself unable to enjoy her legitimate intimate sexual relationship with her husband. This led to frustration and hurt on both sides, and almost ruined their marriage.

Mary had never truly repented of her earlier sin. Believing that the sin of premarital sex compounded by the abortion was just too terrible for God to forgive, she hadn't bothered to ask for forgiveness. As well as being weighed down by guilt and remorse, she was also full of bitterness and resentment as to what might have been. She often dreamed of what it would have been like if that awful night had never happened. By now she might have been a successful lawyer married to Bill who was going to be a doctor. They would have been active in their church; something which she felt she never could be now, because that would be so hypocritical. But here she was, no career, an unhappy marriage and nearly always on anti-depressant pills.

Of course it didn't need to be like that. Not only was she living with the consequences of her past sin but Mary was also successfully allowing her past to ruin her present enjoyment of life. Mary needed, in true repentance, to ask for forgiveness. She could be free of her past but she would have to accept both the consequences of her action in the past and God's forgiveness. She was married now, and it was not to Bill. She wasn't a lawyer, she was a housewife, but that didn't mean that her life needed to be unbearable or even unpleasant. There was forgiveness available and freedom from the guilt and pain of the past. Life could never be as it might have been, but God could make it equally fulfilling and rich.

Making a choice

A sinful act does not take place without warning: it is preceded by a sinful thought which in turn is preceded by desire. James talks about this: 'but each one is tempted when, by his own evil desire, he is dragged away and enticed. Then, after desire has conceived, it gives birth to sin; and sin, when it is full-grown, gives birth to death' (Jas 1:14–15).

It is at the point of desire and thought that we must make our choice about our course of action. Once we have begun to sin it is more difficult to stop and turn back. There is at least a moment of time in which to choose. The wrong choice, although made in only a matter of seconds, may result in a lifetime of regret. For Tom his wrong choice cost him dearly.

Tom had worked his way up the ladder to become a successful business executive. He lived in a lovely house with his wife and three children and enjoyed a comfortable style of living. Tom had been a Christian for a number of years and was the secretary of his church fellowship.

One day at work Tom found himself embarrassingly short of cash. He knew he could put in a false expenses claim and get some money straight away. He could balance it up the next time he had expenses by deducting the appropriate amount. No one would ever know.

The following week Tom was again short of money. They had recently moved to a bigger house with a bigger mortgage and money was very tight at present. It had worked so easily last week with the false expenses claim. Why not do it again? Tom argued with himself, 'It's not really honest, but on the other hand I've worked hard for the firm—why shouldn't they help me out when I'm finding things difficult?' After the first few times it became quite easy for Tom to put in a false claim each week. By doing this he increased his salary by £100 per month tax free. Tom knew full well that what he was doing was wrong, but he quite deliberately kept on sinning. He was living a double life. Publicly he was church secretary and an upright and honest businessman, but secretly he was deliberately stealing from his employers.

One day Tom discovered that the firm's auditors were paying considerable attention to the expenses claim forms. At this Tom broke out in a cold sweat, his heart rate doubled and he felt sick. He suddenly realised the implications of what he had done. How could he have been so foolish? Why had they moved house and put a millstone round their neck (which was what their new mortgage seemed like)? They had been quite happy and comfortable in the previous house, but Catherine wanted a bigger kitchen and he wanted a bigger garden. Why could they not have been content? Now look at the mess he was in.

That night Tom tossed and turned in bed, Catherine asked him what the matter was but he said he was fine. How could he tell her? He might lose his job, and how would he explain that to her and to everyone else? He prayed much that night, asking God to forgive him and not to let anyone find out what he had done. But like David of long ago, Tom was to discover that God will not tolerate the double life. What is done in secret may be exposed openly for all to see: 'You did it in secret, but I will do this thing in broad daylight before all Israel' (2 Sam 12:12).

The following week a very worried and haggard Tom was ushered into the boss's office. Tom was asked to account for all his expenses claims. Of course he couldn't. He broke down, more because of the mounting tension of the previous week of waiting and worrying than anything else. He asked his boss to forgive him and promised to repay all the money. However, Tom's boss took a dim view of dishonesty and Tom was asked to resign.

One of the hardest things for Tom was facing his family and friends. Of course he had to resign as church secretary. Not only had his action hurt himself, but it had caused his family great pain. It had also brought dishonour to the church and most of all to God.

For months afterwards Tom was angry and bitter against God. Why had God let him be found out? God knew he was sorry and could easily have caused things to be hushed up or just not discovered. After all, there must be hundreds of folks filling in false expenses claims. But it had all become so public. Even the local newspaper had run an article on 'the church secretary who was swindling his firm out of money'. Did everyone need to know about it? The shame of it all had almost driven him to commit suicide.

Tom felt abandoned by God. He fluctuated between intense anger at the unfairness of his punishment, and remorse for his own sin. If only he had said no instead of yes to the thought of filling in a false expenses claim all those months back, just to get himself out of a financial problem. The choice had been his; he could blame no one but himself. There were other things he could have done to raise money. They could have cancelled their holiday or sold their car or even moved back to a smaller house. But the temptation was too strong.

Resisting temptation

Was the temptation too strong? Are we mere victims of our circumstances with no power to resist? Can we ever claim a special licence to sin? We have been promised that we will never be tempted above what we are able: 'No temptation has seized you except what is common to man. And God is faithful; he will not let you be tempted beyond what you can bear. But when you are tempted, he will also provide a way out so that you can stand up under it' (1 Cor 10:13).

Can any of us condemn Tom or Mary? Who of us has never yielded to temptation? Our sin may not have had such far-reaching consequences, and for that we should be truly thankful. We are all weak, but recognising our weakness can, in fact, make us strong.

God knows how weak we are and so it was that Jesus frequently told his disciples to watch and pray. In Gethsemane Jesus warned the disciples again: 'Watch and pray so that you will not fall into temptation. The spirit is willing, but the body is weak' (Mt 26:41).

It is probably when we think we are strong that we are most at risk from falling. The devil longs to find us off guard and without the protective armour of watchful prayer, for then we are vulnerable to his enticing temptations. Tom had thought he could sin once and then cover it up. He had thought he was strong but discovered how weak he was.

Paul also knew the need for watchfulness against sin and temptation and told the Corinthians 'So, if you think you are standing firm, be careful that you don't fall!' (1 Cor 10:12) It is only as we stay close to God, recognising how weak we are, and fully dependant on his power and strength, that we can be safe from temptation.

How was Tom going to allow this past sin to affect his life? He could remain bitter and resentful about the harsh treatment he felt he had received. No doubt there were many of his Christian friends who were wrongly judgemental of Tom and unwilling to forgive him. They knew nothing of how often Tom had resisted temptation. Tom had sinned, and God had dealt with him. None of us is sinless: our reaction to Tom's sin should be to see it as a warning that we too can fall into temptation, and we must be constantly and prayerfully on our guard.

An alternative to bitterness was for Tom to remain a broken man; ever conscious of how he had let God and his family and friends down, for ever living in the shadow of his sin, and as a result disqualifying himself from future service to God.

In later years Tom was able to look back on this episode of his life without agonising or crushing pain. He had experienced God's love and knew that no sin, when repented of, could keep him from his Father's love. He came to realise too that it was God's kindness which exposed his sin. Without that exposure Tom would have continued to sin and his spiritual life would have withered and died. When Tom was made to face the consequences of his actions he was brought face to face with a holy God who does not smile benevolently on sin, no matter how inconsequential we consider it. In allowing Tom to lose his job and position in the church God was applying drastic emergency surgery in order to save Tom's life. With God's help Tom was able to rebuild his life. He developed a ministry within the church to people who were struggling with temptation. People felt able to talk to Tom about their own weaknesses and failures because they knew Tom would understand.

There is one more comment to make on this subject of sin. Although sin and failure *can* be a cause of depression, we must never assume that this is always the case. For many, depression is an illness which has as little to do with sin, and the need for forgiveness, as does influenza; and we shall look at this in the next chapter.

8

Stress or Illness?

In times of stress, we tend to resort to behaviour patterns we have learned in the past. The person who reacts in anger when his will is thwarted may completely lose control and strike out in all directions under severe stress. People who have never learned to deal with conflict in their lives will in later life try to avoid it by turning their back on it or even by denying its existence. Those who have never had to (or been allowed to) make decisions in their early life will find decision-making almost impossible under stress. They will try to avoid the issue facing them and will often withdraw into themselves for fear of making the wrong decision.

It is, however, important to distinguish between people who lack confidence because of their past experiences and people who lack confidence because they have a depressive or other form of mental illness. Before deciding that a problem is a spiritual one or caused by the past, we must be sure it is not due to illness. Otherwise we can do great harm and cause much pain.

Clinical depression

Jane was distraught when she phoned me. 'Mr Smith says I should throw all my pills away. He says I don't need pills, I need faith. What can I do? My doctor says I need the pills.'

Jane had been ill for several months and her GP had referred her to a psychiatrist. He had diagnosed a depressive illness and prescribed anti-depressant tablets for her.

Mr Smith was Jane's minister. He did not believe that Christians should get depressed. He certainly didn't believe that they should consult psychiatrists or take pills to help them. If they were unhappy they needed more faith to experience the 'joy of the Lord.' It was little wonder that Jane was distraught. She was caught in the middle of conflicting advice.

Many Christians are bewildered about mental illness, wondering whether or not it is right for Christians to be mentally ill. Many attribute weakness, failure, or lack of faith to those who experience any form of mental illness, but particularly to those who have what many term 'a nervous breakdown' or who suffer a form of depressive illness.

When I was a young student I remember chatting to my minister and asking him whether he felt that Christians should get depressed or not. His reply was a question to me. 'Do you think Christians should get appendicitis?' At the time I remember thinking his response a little odd, but over the years I have come to understand it.

There has always been a social stigma about entering mental hospitals—asylums, as they were once called. With greater understanding of mental illness and better forms of treatment that stigma is diminishing, although it remains to a certain extent. Within Christian popular thinking there is certainly a stigma attached to those who claim to be Christians and require treatment for mental illness.

Ann, a friend of mine, once telephoned me in tears. Her distress was due to the fact that her doctor had told her that she was depressed and required anti-depressant tablets. Ann felt intense shame about this. If her GP had told her she had a serious heart condition she would have coped better with that diagnosis, but to be told that she needed anti-depressants was in Ann's eyes the equivalent of being told she was a hopeless failure as a Christian.

Why is there such reluctance to accept the fact that our minds as well as our bodies are subject to illness from time to time? I think part of the problem lies in differentiating between what is merely an inability to cope with the problems of life and what is genuinely illness.

If we are prepared to accept that Christians become physically unwell then we also have to accept that they can become mentally unwell. When Jane told me of Mr Smith's comments to her I reminded her that Mr Smith was attending his doctor for a form of rheumatism and was taking medicine for that. Why should she not also accept a doctor's advice that she required medicine for her illness?

But the real question was—was Jane ill? If she was ill, then clearly she needed to be treated by the medical profession just like others who are ill. However, if she was not 'ill', then perhaps spiritual counsel would be of more benefit.

Mrs Grey, a 53-year-old mother of three, walked

slowly dragging her feet into her GP's surgery. She sat down as if heaving a great weight into the chair. Her hair was uncombed and her face without make-up, and she looked a picture of misery. When asked what her problem was she shrugged her shoulders and said, 'I don't know. Life doesn't seem worth living. I am such a terrible person. I've made life miserable for all my family. I'm no use to anyone. I can't concentrate and I've lost all my confidence. I used to think I was a Christian but I can't pray, I can't read my Bible and I don't want to go to church. God can't love someone like me. I can't even cry any more. I can't sleep, and I've lost a stone in weight because I can't be bothered eating. I wake early every morning but I don't want to get out of bed because I can't face another day. Mornings are the worst. I can't remember when I last felt happy. I wouldn't have come to see you, but my family said I had to. You can't do anything for me. Nobody can.'

Mrs Grey spoke in a flat, monotonous tone, her face mask-like throughout. After she had said all this she had almost no other spontaneous speech. She was clearly suffering from a depressive illness. A misguided Christian friend had tackled her on her inability to pray, read her Bible and go to church. She had suggested that she had sin in her life of which she needed to repent before she would feel the desire to resume these activities. She had told Mrs Grey how bad she was, but Mrs Grey had merely agreed with her.

Suffering from stress

Angela was lying between the white sheets of a hospital bed looking very sorry for herself. She was recovering from having taken an overdose of her grandmother's sleeping pills. She complained bitterly that she was depressed and nobody was taking any notice of her.

Angela was twenty-six. She had been married for three years to her young, up-and-coming executive husband. He was ambitious, striving to reach the top of his profession. Before they had married Ken had been attentive, caring and considerate. After their marriage they had moved to another town because of Ken's work. Angela had been unable to get a job. She didn't know anyone in the town and felt quite isolated. Ken's driving ambition occupied much of his time. He was more than willing to work overtime, telling Angela that it was the only way to be noticed in his firm. He would never get promotion unless his boss saw his commitment. When he came home at night Ken was tired and irritable. All he wanted to do was collapse in front of the television set while Angela was desperate for someone to speak to.

Angel's feelings toward her husband were ambivalent. She wanted him to do well in his job and gain promotion—he would earn more money then—but she wanted him to spend more time with her. She had an idealised picture of marriage. Her father had not been ambitious; he had worked hard and was content with his position as a bank clerk. His interests were simple and mainly revolved around the home. Angela, the only daughter among four sons, had been indulged by her father—in fact his life had been centred on Angela. Angela could not understand why her husband wanted to have interests apart from her. She wanted to be the very centre of his life, but at present Ken's work seemed to be competing for that place. Ken soon began to feel suffocated by Angela's desire to have all of his attention all of the time. He felt quite inadequate to quench Angela's insatiable appetite. This made him withdraw even more from her, seeking escape in his work which in turn created panic in her.

Angela had once read a book where the heroine had taken an overdose of sleeping pills because she had been jilted by her boyfriend. This act had caused the boyfriend to return to her because he realised how much he loved her. When Angela took her grand-mother's sleeping pills she had no intention of killing herself. In fact she made absolutely sure she would be discovered in time by telephoning her husband at work immediately after taking the pills. Her aim was to make Ken realise the importance of paying attention to her. If he would not listen to her constant nagging he would surely have to take notice of her action.

Consulting an expert

Both Angela and Mrs Grey require help but the kind of help they need is quite different. Mrs Grey requires medical treatment for her obvious depressive illness. That treatment can be undertaken by her own GP who will prescribe anti-depressant tablets. However, her illness is quite severe and she is at far more risk of committing suicide than Angela is. Mrs Grey has lost the desire to live, she feels useless and a bother to everyone. She has a form of mental illness and may require to see a psychiatrist and may need some time as an in-patient in a psychiatric hospital.

It can sometimes be difficult for non-medical people to tell when someone is suffering from depression rather than the transient changes of mood that we all experience. Many of us may have at times in our life felt useless and a bother to folk. So what is the difference? A true medical depression will be intense and unremitting. Often people feel much worse in the mornings but eventually feel bad all day every day. They lose interest in things they used to enjoy, and feel a burden to everyone. Guilt is a common feature, and one which Christians may mistake for conviction of sin. Depressed people have a vague sense of guilt: it is not usually specific. They have a general sense of impending doom which is not open to reason, nor can they be persuaded that there is any help for them or forgiveness for their sin. The guilt is usually unjustified; their families will deny that they have done all the things they accuse themselves of doing. They may claim that they have caused the family shameful disgrace and brought calamity upon them, none of which is true. Christians can cause great pain and harm by entering such a situation with a handful of Christian cliches, exhorting the person to put more trust in God and confess their sin.

Mrs Grey will require spiritual help and support, but her pressing need is to obtain the proper medical treatment. If you came across someone in the street who had fallen and broken his leg, your first priority would be to get the person to a medical centre where his broken leg could be attended to. You wouldn't interrogate him first about his attendance at church or try to discover if he broke his leg as a result of sin rather than misfortune. Whatever the cause, the broken leg requires medical treatment. Similarly, when someone is in mental pain he requires the proper treatment for it. When there is any shadow of doubt about whether medical treatment is necessary, a medical opinion should always be sought. It is like the man with the broken leg. You may not be sure if the leg is broken, but you wouldn't ask him to wait and see. You would seek a medical opinion immediately.

Angela would normally be seen by a psychiatrist before her discharge from hospital. Most patients who are admitted to hospital following an attempted suicide are seen by a psychiatrist before discharge, to assess whether or not it was a genuine suicide attempt, and to see if the patient is suffering from any form of mental illness which requires treatment.

Neurotic symptoms

Angela claimed to be depressed, but what she was feeling was more to do with frustration, loneliness and problems within her marriage. She was displaying what the medical profession call neurotic symptoms. Neurotic symptoms such as anxiety, depression, occasional short-lived obsessional thoughts and physical symptoms without an organic cause are experienced by most people in response to the stressful events of everyday life. Indeed, they are often perfectly normal responses which we need not be ashamed of. A certain amount of anxiety is not only normal in certain circumstances but necessary for peak performance. It is what the student has before an exam or the runner experiences before a major track event. This is known as Yerkes-Dodson's law. We need a little anxiety to enhance performance, but the same law goes on to show that once you exceed a certain amount of anxiety, performance falls off. In other words, a little anxiety is all right and even beneficial in certain circumstances; however, too much will be bad for us.

When these symptoms become intense and out of

proportion to the severity of the cause of the stress, we can call it a neurotic illness or a neurosis. For instance, it would be a perfectly normal reaction to be afraid if you suddenly saw a fierce tiger coming towards you, but it would not be so normal to show terror at seeing a docile cat walking on the other side of the road. Similarly it is quite normal to be a little anxious before an important interview, but it is not normal to be anxious every time you leave your home or every time you walk into a shop.

There are certain times in our life when we are more vulnerable to developing neurotic symptoms. As children we start learning to cope with stressful events from the moment we enter the world. The first time we are hungry and do not find immediate alleviation of this we suffer stress. Gradually we learn to accept a certain amount of stress and how to cope with it. However, there is a limit to how much responsibility children can shoulder, and when they are subjected to more stress than they can handle then they too develop symptoms, such as behaviour problems, bedwetting, or undue shyness.

Adolescence is a time when we are trying to find our identity in life. Our emotions may be more fragile and we may react more than is normal to a stressful situation. It is a time of coping with new types of stresses and we have to learn how to handle them.

Many women find that coping with stress is more difficult just prior to their monthly period. They become more irritable and emotionally fragile. Those women who suffer badly from premenstrual tension find this a very difficult time of the month and find coping with additional stress almost impossible. The menopause is also a difficult time for women when they are more prone to develop neurotic symptoms in response to stress.

After the death of a spouse, depression is normal for a limited time until readjustments are made. After the birth of a baby some women develop varying degrees of depression. Retirement is another vulnerable time as is reaching a particular age for some people. For instance, the single woman who is reaching her fortieth birthday may go through a short-lived crisis time when she has to face the fact that marriage prospects are diminishing.

The fact that there are times when we are more vulnerable to stress and may have brief periods when we feel we are not coping well does not mean that we are mentally ill. We need to recognise what is a normal reaction and not be ashamed of the limitations of our frail humanity, while being able to distinguish this from an illness where the symptoms are more severe and long-lasting.

There is a borderline between normal reaction and illness. Normal symptoms may cross over that line to become exaggerations of normality. It is often at this point that many are confused about whether a person is ill or not. When a symptom is interfering severely with a person's ability to lead a normal life, or affecting other people's ability to live with him, then we may consider the symptom to be part of a neurosis. Again, when in doubt, a medical opinion should be sought.

It may not be any major stressful event which tips the balance in favour of illness, but rather a great number of more minor stressful events which are not coped with and dealt with at the time but are allowed to accumulate.

Coping with stress

Many Christians are so ashamed of having any kind of psychological problem, seeing it as weakness, that they do not seek help until they reach the point where they are seriously ill and require specialist help. Many problems, if helped in the early stages, can be prevented from becoming serious. Other Christians, knowing that they have a problem, may approach a Christian friend or even pastor for help, only to be told they need to confess their sin, or have more faith, or receive the baptism of the Spirit or other similar spiritual platitudes. Some of these things may well be true, but people who are struggling with deep psychological problems need much more than that. They need practical guidance about how to deal with their problems, they need reassurance and love, they need support in their struggle, and they may require the specialist help of a psychiatrist or clinical psychologist.

As a Christian, Angela thought she should be able to cope with the isolation and loneliness of her new situation. She knew she wasn't coping but was too ashamed to admit it at first. There were problems in their marriage which again both Angela and Ken were ashamed to admit, even to themselves. 'Surely your marriage will succeed if you marry another Christian! Christians aren't supposed to have problems!' This denial situation went on until Angela reached crisis point, and rational thinking was abandoned because she had to communicate her need of help in the only way she could. Angela doesn't need the help of a psychiatrist. She needs friendship and acceptance in her local church, but most of all she and her husband need some good marital counselling. This could be undertaken by their pastor if he is experienced in that area. With the ever-increasing breakdown of marriage in our society, both secular and Christian, that kind of expertise is essential in the ministry.

'It is impossible to live without stress. Every situation is loaded with it. Stress now contributes to 90 per cent of all illnesses, and half of all visits to the doctor are stress-related.' So writes Rowland Croucher in *Landmarc New Year 1987* published by MARC Europe. Preventive medicine is the best kind, and we can certainly prevent much of the illness caused by stress. We need to learn better methods of coping with stress, and the process may require us to unlearn many maladaptive behaviour patterns which we have learned in the past. We should not be ashamed to admit that we need help. Christians are not immune from the effects of stress in their lives. We are all affected by our past patterns of behaviour and how we have learned to react to stress.

There are, however, some illnesses which are not so easily prevented. Mrs Grey's illness was not a direct result of stress. It is wrong to assume that all Christians will remain free from all mental illness, for there are different forms of mental illness just as there are many kinds of physical illness. Some mental illness has been shown to have a strong genetic component—such as schizophrenia, manic depression, and certain types of depression. Studies have shown that there are various chemicals in the brain which get out of balance, and medication is aimed at restoring the balance. These types of mental illnesses and others such as the dementias and obsessive, compulsive neuroses should always be assessed by someone in the medical profession, usually a psychiatrist, and there should be as much shame attached to them as is attached to having a heart attack.

Christian psychiatrists

I have often heard the comment 'It would be good if there were more Christian psychiatrists because Christians who are mentally ill really need to see a Christian psychiatrist.' While I agree that it would be good to have more Christian psychiatrists, I do not agree with the reason. Christians are urged by Christ to be light and salt in the world and we certainly need Christians to have that effect in the world of psychiatry as in the world of teaching and every other sphere of living.

However, in comparing with most other Christian psychiatrists, I would not agree that Christians who are mentally ill need necessarily see a *Christian* psychiatrist.

I understand why lay people think this way. Our lives have a spiritual dimension which the non-Christian psychiatrist will not be able to understand. However, it is not our spiritual lives that he will be treating, and any good psychiatrist can treat a Christian patient just as well as a Christian psychiatrist. What matters is to see a psychiatrist who is well thought of and highly regarded by his colleagues and has a good track record of success in treating the mentally ill.

We do not say that all Christians must have a Christian GP or see a Christian cardiologist when ill. In some situations it may be an added bonus to find that our doctor is a Christian, but that should not detract from the ability of the non-Christian to do his job as well as, and sometimes better than, a Christian doctor.

Physical and mental illness are part of our inheritance from Adam, and although in Christ we are new creatures, we are still subject to the effects of the world in which we live.

We need to look carefully at the ways in which, with God's help, we can begin to change the parts of our character and personality which hinder our Christian growth and development, while at the same time recognising and accepting illness when it is present. God wants us to take action, whether that involves going to see a doctor when we are ill or striving to learn better ways of dealing with stress.

9

An Instant Cure—or Hard Work?

As a young Christian I came under the influence of a particular type of 'holiness' teaching. I was taught that sanctification was something I had to experience in the same way as I had experienced justification and conversion. At a convention I attended I listened to the preacher waxing eloquent on the need for a sanctification experience. At the end of his talk he asked if there were any present who were dissatisfied with their Christian lives. Were there any who wanted to be more holy, who wanted rid of many of the things in their lives of which they were ashamed?

As I sat listening, my heart said 'yes' to all his questions. I was all too aware of the shortcomings in my Christian life. There was my fierce fiery temper for a start: how I longed to be free of that. I knew I wasn't always as kind and pleasant to people as I should be. Oh, to be all that the preacher said I could be!

Then the preacher asked those who had responded with, 'Yes' in their hearts to come forward for sanctification. Was it really that easy? Could a few short steps to the front of the church really change my whole personality? I was more than willing to try. The preacher prayed with us and I felt a surge of excitement and anticipation. The desire to be all that God wanted me to be was real, but I had never known it was this easy to achieve. Or was it?

For the next few days I walked, or rather floated, around with an air of spiritual piety and if truth be known an air of superiority. I had something other Christians didn't have. I hadn't been able to understand why the whole audience hadn't gone forward for sanctification. Perhaps they already had it—although I knew most of my friends couldn't, for their lives were far from perfect.

About a week later the bubble burst. I was annoyed with my brother over something very trivial and before I knew what was happening, there I was shouting at him. I was cut to the core with shame and disappointment. The very thing I had gone forward for sanctification for—to be more self-controlled and be rid of my bad temper. As the weeks went by I realised that I hadn't changed. What had gone wrong? Had it not worked? Surely God hadn't doubted my sincerity.

A year later at a similar convention I went forward again for sanctification, only to be disappointed a second time. That was almost twenty years ago, and I have long since learned that sanctification is a life-long process of being conformed to the image of Christ. A process which involves me actively, it is not a passive experience.

But the defect lies here: sanctification is rather expected than worked for; rather anticipated as the necessary growth of the germ implanted in regeneration than a development dependant on positive cultivation on the part of man, and on positive energies distinctly and designedly put forth on the part of the great efficient agent, the Holy Ghost.[1]

In justification our works have no place at all and simple faith in Christ is the one thing needful. In sanctification our own works are of vast importance, and God bids us fight and watch and pray and strive and take pains and labour.

Sanctification is eminently a progressive work, and admits of continual growth and enlargement so long as a man lives.[2]

In previous chapters I have tried to demonstrate that what we are and how we behave in the present is largely determined by our past. We inherit from our parents certain characteristics, including some tendencies towards certain temperaments. Children are not born as blank sheets of paper on which the environment begins to write and map out their whole personality. However, neither are we born with our personality fully formed and unchangeable.

The trap which many fall into when considering their personality defects is the same as that into which I fell regarding sanctification. (In fact sanctification involves changing those aspects of our personality which cause both ourselves and others offence.) Many expect an overnight cure or some other form of magic answer to their problems.

God does not change you by magic. No wand will be waved over your head so that your deepest problems vanish overnight. There may be breakthroughs, sudden insights, glorious experiences. But the major work of transformation will be slow and often deeply painful. Yet the pain is immeasurably reduced by trust and understanding.[3]

There is no doubt that we may experience crisis times when God's presence is especially felt and we are convicted in particular areas of our lives. The work of the Holy Spirit is to shine God's light into our lives, focussing on areas which need to be changed. God gives us the desire and grace to change. The power to change also comes from God but it does not work automatically. We need to apply the antiseptic to our wounded lives—and just as antiseptic causes initial pain on an open wound, so we often experience pain in the healing process.

Dealing with the past

How do we work through becoming free from the past, for work we must? I must emphasise here that when I talk of being free from the past I am talking of being free from the binding chains of the past which hold us prisoners, the chains which prevent us from growing in Christ as we should, from reaching our fullest usefulness to God and from enjoying the fullness of life in Christ which we are told we can expect as Christians. We cannot cut ourselves off from the past and pretend it never happened. Our past is part of us and will continue to influence how we think and behave in the present. However, God does not intend us to be prisoners to our past. There are many people, including Christians, who are so tied up in the past that they cannot move forward in the present. It is freedom from that kind of bondage that I am talking about.

A prerequisite for dealing with the past is a wholehearted desire to do so. Of course, before we can have a desire for change we have to recognise the need for change. It would seem incredible that any Christian would not recognise at least one if not many areas of his life which need to be changed for the better. However, if we are blinded by the lies of the devil, telling us that our past and its effect on us is permanent and cannot be changed, then we will settle down to live with it. What is the point of working to effect a change in our lives if we accept that change is impossible? If change is impossible then we need not even try to change.

On the other hand, if we believe that change in our lives happens as a passive event, without any need for our co-operation, then we will see no need for effort on our part. If change does not happen in some magical kind of way then it is not going to happen at all, and we decide to accept our lot in life. Too bad about the past. This is the perfect kind of soil for the seeds of bitterness to grow. For we blame our past for our inability to enjoy the present, and we blame God for allowing our past.

Whatever the cost

There are others who see the need to change, the need to delve into past events and face up to them and they say that they want to change. They may talk of this desire in strong language recounting days and nights spent in prayer about it. No one could doubt their sincerity. The problem is that although they want to change they want to do so on their own terms.

Many go along to see a counsellor, pastor, doctor or friend seeking help. However, when that person starts asking awkward questions the shutters go up. Or when suggestions are made for changes which are unacceptable, the help offered is refused.

You see, many want to change, but without any kind

of upset or inconvenience in their lives. When we say we want to change or be free we need to add 'whatever the cost'. When we come to Jesus and ask for his help in dealing with our personality or our past we need to give him a completely free hand in our lives and be prepared for a certain amount of pain. There are no 'spiritual gains without pains'.

Esther was an example of this kind of person. She had suffered a great deal as a child and this had left many scars, one of which was an inability to mix with large crowds of people. This greatly affected her life. It limited the places she could go to and kept her from attending church. Whenever she went into a large crowd her face went red and her heart rate increased, giving her an uncomfortable feeling in her chest, and then she would begin to have difficulty breathing. In other words, she had a panic attack. This is not an uncommon problem, and is quite easy to treat, but it involves working through the problem and enduring some uncomfortable physical sensations for a time. But Esther was not prepared to tolerate any discomfort, and at the first signs of her heart rate increasing she would immediately retreat from the scene. She kept on blaming her past for the way she was, and in fact used it as an excuse for abandoning the treatment programme. Esther had become used to her 'sick role' and received considerable gain from it. She was able to avoid places she didn't really want to go to, and she had a great deal of attention paid to her—although she always insisted that she didn't like or want attention.

There was no doubt that Esther needed help, and superficially she wanted help, but on her own terms. It had to be the kind of help which didn't require too much from her, involved no pain or discomfort and didn't remove her 'sick role'. Her ability to blame the past for everything which was hindering her Christian growth was very convenient.

'Cast away for ever the vain thought that if a believer does not grow in grace it is not his fault. Settle it in your mind that a believer, a man quickened by the spirit, is not a mere dead creature, but a being of mighty capacities and responsibilities.'[4]

Where our past is interfering with our spiritual growth we have to be prepared to let go of the past. I don't mean we are to pretend it didn't happen, but rather we must actively let go of it. It is all too easy to hug it to ourselves, to nurse it and feed the flames of anger and passion surrounding it. Our past is an all too easy excuse for our unacceptable behaviour.

How do we let go of the past? Like any other problem in our lives we first of all need to grasp the thorn that is our past (thorns are painful things to grasp) and deal with it. The power and grace to do so will be given to us from God, but we need to grapple with it regardless of the pain.

We may need to forgive someone even if they haven't asked for it. Bitterness is a poison which results in slow death.

We need to stop comparing our past with that of others. 'If only I had parents like Susan's I wouldn't have all these problems.' 'If only my mother hadn't died when I was so young and I had two loving parents like John.' 'Mike wasn't ill when he was young, how does he know what it is like to have missed so much school?' 'Jim's wife never ran off and left him for another man; no wonder he can be so happy.' 'Alison's husband doesn't go into rages the way mine does, no wonder I'm a nervous wreck and she is so composed.'

When we get involved in this kind of comparing, what we are saying is, 'God, it's not fair. Why are the circumstances of my life so awful compared to everyone else? It's no wonder I am the way I am. It's all your fault really, not mine.'

God will not erase our past. He doesn't want to erase it, but rather he wants us to learn from it and benefit from it. But he wants us also to walk away from our past taking the lessons learnt but leaving the rest behind. We can't go around dragging our past with us and expect to be free to enjoy the present. Yes, we accept that many terrible things may have happened to us in the past but are they to go on destroying us? Do we need to allow the pain of the past to reach its cold fingers into the present and tarnish all that is good there?

What about the memories, the painful memories? We have two choices. We can either starve these memories so that they shrink and die, or we can feed them to keep them alive and even allow them to grow.

Taking action

Paul's exhortation to the Philippians sheds some light on how this is possible:

> whatever is true, whatever is noble, whatever is right, whatever is pure, whatever is lovely, whatever is admirable—if anything is excellent or praiseworthy—think about such things. Whatever you have learned or received or heard from me, or seen in me—put it into practice. And the God of peace will be with you (Phil 4:8–9).

There are three things in these verses which help us. They are all active. First we are to fill our minds with good things. This is an act of the will, for good things do not always come naturally into our minds. We need to train our minds to think of good rather than bad things. If we are the kind of person who always sees something to criticise, then we need to make a point of looking for things to praise. Dwelling on the past and constantly thinking of and reliving the pain it caused will only feed the memories. We need actively to resist the memories and replace them with the kind of thoughts Paul encourages us to think. The more we do this, hard though it is to begin with, we will find to our amazement that eventually this becomes the pattern of our thinking rather than the other more negative way. Like everything else, with practice it becomes easier.

The next thing Paul encourages us to do is to learn from him. We are to observe others more mature than ourselves and learn from them. We are to take Paul as an example just as he took Jesus as his, and ultimately so do we. This again is an active process, for we do not learn in a passive way: it involves work. If you think back to your school days and trying to learn history or geography, you will recall going over and over the material in order to remember it. One reading was seldom enough, for learning is a continuing process. Similarly, when dealing with our past simply saying, 'Right, that's it, I'm going to put the past behind me' will not result in an immediate solution. You may need help. Just as a pupil needs help from a teacher, so you may need help from an experienced counsellor, friend or doctor in learning how to deal with your past. You may need to learn the lessons several times. You may need to look hard to see what you can learn from your past rather than dwelling on all the harmful effects of it. It will take time and effort and not a little pain.

The third thing which Paul tell us to do (for he is, through the Holy Spirit, speaking to us as well as to the Philippians) is to put into practice what we have learnt. Nothing passive about that. This is undoubtedly the hardest part. It is one thing to know what is wrong and how to put it right, but quite another actually to put this into practice. This is very often the painful part and the place where many decide that the terms of getting better or being free from the past are too costly. For Esther it meant giving up her 'sick role', gradually learning to mix with people and suffering a few minutes of discomfort—she had been taught how to control her panic attack, but putting this into practice involved some discomfort to begin with. It involved learning to be interested in other people, learning new topics of conversation other than her traumatic past and subsequent difficulties, and it involved trusting God for her future. For Esther the cost of getting better was too great.

There are many different reasons why people hang on to their past, but in doing so they are denying themselves the full joy of the present. They will never reach their full potential in terms of what they can be and achieve for God, or know the full depth of peace which he offers us.

Forgive me quoting from J C Ryle again, but he was a man of great wisdom and I have found his writings of great benefit:

> This paper may fall into the hands of some who ought to know something of growth in grace, but at present know nothing at all. They have made little or no progress since they were first converted. They have "settled on their lees" (Zeph 1:12). They go on from year to year content with old grace, old experience, old knowledge, old faith,

old measure of attainment, old religious expressions, old set phrases. Like the Gibeonites, their bread is always mouldy and their shoes are patched and clouted. They never appear to get on. Are you one of these people? If you are, you are living far below your privileges and responsibilities. It is high time to examine yourself.[5]

We can know freedom to enjoy God and all his rich blessings without the shadow of the past hanging over us and preventing the rays of his sunshine penetrating deep into our hearts. But there is no instant cure, and we need to work at it.

10

Low Self-esteem

Lack of confidence and low self-esteem are common problems and their cause can be clearly linked to the sufferer's past. If these traits are present in our personality they hinder our growth as Christians, affect our willingness to serve God for fear of failure, and restrict our enjoyment of the present.

Childhood experiences

In an attempt to break a child's will and make him more obedient and compliant, many parents make the mistake of attacking the child instead of the child's behaviour. For instance, little Johnny has just tried to help in the kitchen by putting the milk in the fridge but he is really too small to reach the right shelf for it. In his struggle he drops the milk and spills it all over the newly washed kitchen floor. That is enough to make most mums upset. Unfortunately this is not the first time this has happened: Johnny is always trying to help but his mum really wishes he wouldn't bother because it always ends up creating more work for her.

There are two responses here. One is that Mum grabs Johnny by the scruff of the neck and shakes him.

'You stupid boy. How many times do I have to tell you not to do that? Don't try to help me again. You are a useless clumsy horrible boy. Look at the floor. I will have to spend ages cleaning it. Go away.'

The other response is that Mum is equally annoyed and upset but says, 'Johnny, look what you have done. That was a silly thing to do. Why didn't you wait until I could help you? I appreciate your trying to help, you are a very kind and helpful boy and Mummy loves you very much, but there are some things that you are still too little to do. Next year when you have grown a little more you will be able to put the milk away, but until then why don't you just put the butter in the fridge for Mummy? Now go and get the mop and you can help me clean up.'

The first response is attacking Johnny as a person, attacking his sense of self-worth. It is Johnny who is useless, clumsy and horrible. His help is not wanted, in fact Mummy tells him to go away. In the next response Mummy is probably just as upset, but she attacks the thing that Johnny has done rather than Johnny himself. There is a subtle but important difference. Mummy reassures Johnny that he is still valued and so is his help (demonstrated by asking for his help to clean up). She still gets the message over that she does not want Johnny to put the milk away, but gives him something else to do instead.

If a child grows up in an environment where his sense of self-worth is constantly being attacked and devalued, where his help is never good enough and he feels unwanted, then he will almost inevitably suffer from low self-esteem as an adult.

There are other ways in which our self-esteem can be damaged. Teachers can contribute to it in school by openly criticising pupils and their work without ever encouraging or praising them. Children are very easily embarrassed, and peer acceptance is important. Being ridiculed in front of friends and classmates can be devastating to young children. As children our sense of self-worth is fragile, and it comes from being valued by those adults closest to us. When the important adults in our young lives refuse to show that they value us and our opinion, we grow up with the feeling that we are not important and don't have anything worthwhile to say or do.

Worth in God's eyes

How does low self-esteem manifest itself in adults? Usually it is seen in a lack of confidence, an inability to make decisions for fear that we are wrong. Sometimes adults try too hard to impress people, believing that just being themselves would never be sufficient. They don't *feel* important and so believe themselves to be thought unimportant by others.

If we fit that description how do we cope with it? Our past experiences have made us this way. Can we undo the harm? The message of the last chapter was that there are no easy answers to our problems. They will not vanish as if by magic. But with God's help, and effort on our part we can work through most of our problems and I believe the same is true of low self-esteem.

Part of the problem in low self-esteem is that our perception of ourselves is wrong. How we perceive ourselves, how others perceive us and how God perceives us are often quite different. So the first thing is to try and get our perception of ourselves more in line with God's perception of us, because his is the only true one.

If we have grown up being told by deed and word that we have little or no value then it will be difficult to believe that anybody, even God, could see any value in us. This is where being a Christian is of tremendous advantage, for we have the scriptures containing God's message for us and this must be our starting point.

'Look at the birds of the air; they do not sow or reap or store away in barns, yet your heavenly Father feeds them. Are you not much more valuable than they?' (Mt 6:26)

The whole message of the scriptures is that we are of such worth to God that he sent his only Son into the world to die for us so that our relationship with God could be restored. Why? Because he wants us, he loves us, he values us, and there are no exceptions. We need to let that message sink deep into our hearts.

The scriptures also tell us that God wants us to be his servants, to serve him in the world. Because of our low self-esteem and our wrong perception of ourselves we feel useless and our help of little value. We may also have a wrong perception of what constitutes valuable service. It is not only the person who preaches God's word or the missionary who goes overseas who is doing valuable service to God. Befriending the lonely, encouraging those who are downcast, making a cup of tea for someone in need—these are all valuable in God's eyes. Whatever we do, if we do it to God's glory, he is well pleased with us. Sweeping out the church and making it ready for Sunday worship if done in God's name, and for his glory, is equally as important as proclaiming God's word to his people. Do we really believe that? In this age of rewards for paper qualifications and high achievements it is difficult not to be influenced by this way of evaluating people. Remember that God's way of assessing us is to look into our hearts, not at what we do, but at what we are before him.

If we made a list of all the people in our church who we thought were important, and then were able to compare it with God's list, I believe we would get quite a surprise. 'But the Lord said to Samuel, "Do not consider his appearance or his height, for I have rejected him. The Lord does not look at the things man looks at. Man looks at the outward appearance, but the Lord looks at the heart"' (1 Sam 16:7).

Every redeemed sinner is of such value to God that he has adopted us into his family and calls us sons and daughters. My husband and I have adopted three children and so the whole image of adoption is a familiar one to us. We took each child into our home and legally made them our own. In the sight of the law it is as if they had been born to us. We are legally responsible for them and they are our heirs. We treat them as if we had conceived and given birth to them. They are important to us and stand in a very special relationship to us; we are their parents. They belong to us in every way and we love them. God has adopted us; we belong to him through Christ.

We may not think that there is much that we can do to advance the kingdom of God. But consider these verses from Matthew's Gospel:

For I was hungry and you gave me something to eat, I was thirsty and you gave me something to drink, I was a stranger and you invited me in, I needed clothes and you clothed me, I was sick and you looked after me, I was in prison and you came to visit me (Mt 25:35).

I tell you the truth, whatever you did for one of the least of these brothers of mine, you did for me (Mt 25:40).

God will never ask more of us than we are able to do. We need to meditate on and digest the scriptures and take to ourselves the worth which God bestows on us.

Once we have laid a firm foundation in our lives of the facts of biblical truth that convince us of our value and worth, regardless of whatever we may feel about ourselves, there is much on a day-to-day practical level that we can do to help ourselves overcome our handicap.

Building up confidence

A 'right' marriage can do much to help us if we suffer from low self-esteem, but a 'wrong' marriage can underline and increase it. If we have a marriage partner who is able to encourage us in all the little things we do and give us praise when appropriate, our confidence will get a chance to grow. However, we may be unfortunate enough to have a marriage partner who is constantly critical of us, always putting us down (especially publicly), enjoying jokes at our expense and never satisfied with anything we do. This is effectively a continuation of our childhood environment which constantly attacks our sense of self worth.

We need to communicate to our spouses the effect they are having on us, either good or bad. The good spouse should be thanked and told how much he or she is helping and this will encourage them to continue and even look for other ways of helping increase our self confidence. The bad spouse needs to be confronted and told that this behaviour is not acceptable and indeed harmful. If you stand up to your spouse in this way you may be amazed to discover that he or she respects you more for it.

Be aware of the effect you have on other people. People with low self-esteem need praise and encouragement, but their behaviour at times can make them unattractive. Their retiring, self-depreciating manner can alienate them from others and be misinterpreted as stand-offish. It can be very tiresome to be with people who are constantly apologising for themselves and their work. Their constant need for reassurance can be off-putting to the very people they crave praise from. Their indecisiveness, due to lack of confidence in their ability, can make them seem unreliable. They may say 'Yes' when asked to do something or go somewhere, but then later feel inadequate for the task and cry off.

How do you overcome this? Forget about what other people think of you. You are God's child, and he is pleased with you. In the words of the Puritan writer Thomas Watson you are the 'blood royal of Heaven'.[1] Whenever you find yourself apologising, check to see whether an apology is really necessary or appropriate. Stop complaining that you are useless. Discover what you are good at and develop that talent. If you are good at noticing new faces in the church congregation, make sure you welcome them and see that as one of your acts of service. Have you time to pray for all the house-bound people in your church? Are you good at baking for the coffee morning? It doesn't need to be anything big. Start small and build up your confidence.

It is possible to increase our confidence by setting ourselves small tasks. Start with something simple and easy so that you are sure of success. Each success is an encouragement to go on and try something else. If you set yourself an unrealistic task then the chances of failure are greater, resulting in disappointment and discouragement and an unwillingness to try anything else.

For instance, if you are very shy about going into crowded places and meeting new people, start off with somewhere you know. Decide that you will go along and take the initiative in one conversation: in other words, you are going to go up to one person and speak to him. Rehearse what you think you could say. Pick something you have heard about on the news, or ask the person something about himself. Don't be put off if he doesn't respond in the way you would like; the important thing is that you did it. You went up to someone and spoke to him. Keep doing this in an environment in which you are familiar, possibly your church, until you feel happy about doing it. Then set yourself a slightly more difficult task and keep at that until you feel happy. It is hard work and initially you may feel very self conscious, but I can assure you that if you persevere you will be successful. It is a good idea to share what you are doing with someone you trust who can help you and certainly pray for you.

Ultimately our self-confidence and sense of worth and value as Christians comes from our confidence in God and our relationship with him. The Queen's children derive their importance from the fact that they are her children rather than anyone else's. We are God's children, the King of kings and Lord of lords, the Creator of the universe. We have no need to be ashamed. God has bestowed on us the inestimable privilege of being his children.

II

Psychotherapy for Christians?

We have seen that Christians are not immune from the
damaging effects of some of their past experiences—
but where does the Christian go for help? There is a
great deal of suspicion about psychiatrists and psychologists. Is it justified? When it comes to dealing with
our past do psychiatrists have all the answers? They
certainly have a great deal to say about how our past
affects us.

I have recently spent two years as a registrar in
psychiatry, and during my training I was involved in
learning about psychotherapy and psychoanalysis. Both
of these disciplines are particularly involved in studying
our past and how it affects our present behaviour.

Many laymen think that most psychiatrists practise
psychodynamic psychotherapy. They imagine that
almost every patient who goes to see a psychiatrist lies
on a couch while the psychiatrist probes deep into the
patient's mind and past. This is simply not true: in fact,
it is extremely difficult to obtain this kind of treatment
on the NHS. Only a few psychiatrists go on to train in
psychoanalysis and psychotherapy.

Psychotherapy is a less intense form of treatment
than psychoanalysis. During psychoanalysis a patient

will attend for treatment up to five times per week for up to five years: this kind of treatment is rarely if ever available on the NHS. For psychotherapy, on the other hand, a patient will normally attend only once a week for perhaps six months to two years.

However, all psychiatrists learn the principles and history of psychoanalysis and psychotherapy during their general training. Therefore they use some of this background knowledge in their general psychiatric treatment.

Theories of psychiatry

Many lay people are confused by what they hear about people like Freud and Jung and so I think it is helpful briefly to consider some of the teaching of the well-known psychiatrists and psychoanalysts.

When I first began my studies, what struck me most was the variety of schools of thought, and within these the further differences of opinion. Practising psychotherapists belong to different schools of thought depending on whom they studied under, although they still bring to their treatment sessions their own views, developed from their own experience of patients.

We cannot go into the details of all the different schools of thought, but rather we will take time to look at the variety of opinion within these schools and at some of the men and women who formed them.

Freud, the father of psychoanalysis, believed that religion was a mass delusion. This is how he viewed religion:

> Religion represents the externalisation of man's unconscious conflicts and their raising to the cosmic level. In one of its aspects it provides substitute gratification for primi-

tive drives, in another it acts as a suppressive force against primitive drives. Religion is "the universal neurosis of humanity" in which is perpetuated the illusion of a loving heavenly Father who promises happiness in the hereafter in return for the renunciation of instinctual drives on earth...When the inhibiting forces of civilisation are removed, however, we see men in their true light, as "savage beasts to whom the thought of sparing their own kind is alien."[1]

Freud's view of man and of religion obviously influenced his teaching of psychoanalysis. I know of no formal school of psychotherapy or psychoanalysis which views man as created in the image of God.

There are of course other famous names in psychoanalysis: Jung, Otto Rank, Melanie Klein, Adler, Karen Horney, Anna Freud, Fairbairn, Erich Fromm, Harry Stack Sullivan and many others. The amazing thing is all of them have their own particular theories, which they believe to be right but which are impossible to prove.

Otto Rank (1884–1939), an Austrian, believed that all neurosis originates in the trauma of birth. Separation from one's mother at birth produces anxiety which in later years may be reactivated by other separation experiences. There are others who predate the problems we have in the present to the prenatal period.

Freud's name is associated with the Oedipus complex and the division of the personality into the super ego, the ego and the id. Many of his theories were to do with sexual relationships.

Melanie Klein believed that babies perceive the world in terms of good and bad objects. The breast which gives milk is a good object while the mother who scolds or withholds milk or food is a bad object. 'Good objects' are taken in or introjected by the child, while 'bad objects' are projected. This process helps to form the child's personality. She worked mainly with children and attempted psychotherapy with children as young as two years old.

Alfred Adler started out as a follower of Freud's theories but later departed from them. Adler believed that neurosis was an attempt to free oneself from feelings of inferiority so as to gain a feeling of superiority. He also believed in the importance of cultural factors which Melanie Klein tended to dismiss.

It is to Jung that we owe the commonly used words 'introvert' and 'extrovert'. J A C Brown has this to say about Jung, who is probably best known in lay circles for his work on dream interpretation:

> Having a wide knowledge of the religion, philosophy, myths, and symbolism of many cultures, Jung has made full use of this knowledge in the psychology—so much so, that many critics have commented that the Jungian theory is more like a metaphysical system than a school of Scientific psychology.[2]

Karen Horney did not agree with Freud's concept of the libido and death instinct, and indeed rejected them. She believed the 'real self' was at the core of human personality, and that healthy growth involved self-realisation as well as the ability to deal with anxiety.

I trust I have said enough to show the diversity of opinion. Indeed, Charles Ryecroft, in his introduction to his book, *A Critical Dictionary of Psychoanalysis*, says this:

> It is a notorious and melancholy fact that psychoanalysts lack the capacity to agree among themselves and that their professional organisations exhibit an apparently inherent tendency towards fission. Their disruptive controversies are typically not of the minor, technical kind which occur

in every science and branch of medicine, but concern fundamental principles, even though they are often found to involve clashes of personality and temperament when viewed historically.

A different view of man

However, there is one theme which I believe is common to many of these theories, and that is the concept of determinism. This theory suggests that our personality is determined by our past, and there is no room for God or his influence.

The aim of psychotherapy is not to make you a better, kinder or even nicer person; indeed, the personal histories of many of the analysts themselves bear out that fact. Rather the aim seems to be to help one to cope with and accept oneself. The psychiatrist will not attempt to reorientate a homosexual so that he becomes heterosexual, but rather he will attempt to help the homosexual accept himself as he is. The aim is to help him to rid himself of guilt feelings and find ways of enjoying life as he is.

It is difficult wholly to embrace a system which is founded on such a completely different view of man and God from that held by Christians.

Christians believe that God is Lord and master of their lives. Humanists believe that man is his own lord and master. As Christians we look to God for strength and grace: our confidence is in his power, in his ability to help us. Humanists believe that strength comes from within themselves and lean on their own ability to help themselves. Indeed, a cult of selfism has sprung up from this kind of teaching.

Guilt is another problem for the humanist, who sees

it as something to be got rid of. Sin and the need for forgiveness are alien concepts for the humanist, whereas they are central to the Christian gospel.

It is difficult, therefore, to see how Christians can be helped in dealing with their past using a form of treatment, whether psychotherapy or psychoanalysis, which is based on a value system so different from the one on which Christians base their whole lives.

I must make it clear that I am not dismissing psychiatrists or even psychotherapy. Many of the insights and techniques they use can help our own understanding of how the past has affected us, and how to move towards restoration, healing and freedom.

I have already taken great pains to show earlier on that Christians who are mentally *ill* should feel no shame in consulting a psychiatrist. Psychiatrists are doctors who have specialised in the branch of medicine dealing with mental illness, and as such should be valued by us. But we are now dealing here with psychological problems which seem related to past experiences, not to illness.

Am I, therefore, saying that there is no place for Christians having psychotherapy? I do not feel that I am in a position to advise either in favour of or against. What I would say is that we need to be aware of the different value system held by many psychotherapists. However, there is much in their skill as doctors, and as men and women experienced in dealing with problems related to our past, from which we can benefit. I have known Christians with deep emotional problems caused by a traumatic past who have found psychotherapy extremely helpful in understanding themselves and how their past has affected them. They have received great benefit from this form of treatment and have been enabled to find release from their past as a result.

A Christian frame of reference

I have many psychiatrist and psychologist friends and colleagues to whom I would not hesitate to recommend Christians. However, we cannot expect the psychiatrist or psychotherapist to guide us in the realm of moral or ethical issues or help us with what are essentially spiritual problems. We do not expect this of doctors in other fields of medicine, nor should we expect it of the psychiatrist. Indeed, any good psychiatrist will make this plain to his patient and will not try to take on a role which is not rightfully his.

There may be other psychiatrists, however, who allow their own value system to influence their treatment of the patient, and Christians should be aware of this. This does apply more to situations where the psychiatrist is using psychotherapy or psychoanalysis as a form of treatment. However, any good psychotherapist would again recognise his own limitations and would not presume to advise a patient to act against his own religious beliefs or moral code. As in every walk of life we get those in the profession of psychiatry and psychology who, although having the same qualification, are not very good at their job.

I have known a case where a young woman engaged to be married attended a psychologist for treatment of a sexual problem rooted in past sexual abuse. The girl was a Christian and did not want to enter into the sexual act with her fiancé before her marriage to him. Even so the psychologist, knowing of the patient's reluctance because of her Christian beliefs, strongly recommended that the girl did so, even to the point of saying that treatment would be discontinued unless she did. The cost of accepting this form of treatment was to be at the expense of this young woman's Christian belief. She rightly recognised this as unacceptable.

I have known others told by psychiatrists that they went to church too much and that that was their real problem. Others were told that what they needed was a sexual experience.

Christians can become too dependent on what their psychiatrist says. This is particularly true in psychotherapy, which involves seeing the therapist at least once a week for perhaps a year or two and maybe more. There are undoubtedly some Christians so scarred by their past that they need the help of a trained person to enable them to be free of it. I believe, though, that when one does embark on such an intense and extended form of treatment one should also have spiritual help and guidance running concurrently. It is often the case that the patient becomes very emotionally involved with the therapist and it is all too easy to allow the therapist to replace God, although the Christian patient would deny this firmly. This is the rationale for concurrent spiritual guidance, as a Christian frame of reference by which to monitor the treatment. We can place too much weight on what the therapist says—after all, he is only working with his own brand of theory.

If it becomes necessary for Christians to have psychotherapy then they should do it prayerfully, seeing the therapist simply as an instrument in God's hands to help them. Ultimately any real help in being free of the past must come from God.

In conclusion, there is most definitely a place for

Christians to consult psychiatrists or psychologists for treatment and help. However, we must be aware of their limitations and not expect them to be our spiritual advisers: for that we must look elsewhere.

12

God's Family

Great is the condescension and mercy which Christ exhibits in building His church! He often chooses the most unlikely and roughest stones, and fits them into a most excellent work. He despises none, and rejects none, on account of former sins and past transgressions. He often makes Pharisees and publicans become the pillars of His house. He delights to show mercy. He often takes the most thoughtless and ungodly, and transforms them into polished corners of His spiritual temple.[1]

How difficult it is for those who are strong to bear with those who are weak, and yet when Jesus lived on earth it was the weak that he seemed particularly interested in. He never sent anyone away on the grounds of their lack of wealth, health or upright moral behaviour. And yet in many of our churches today it is the wealthy, the healthy and apparently 'good' people who are given prominence and importance. There is often an intolerance of weakness. I remember a Christian friend who is active in Christian service, speaking in a derogatory manner of someone who just never seemed to be able to cope with life. Her comment was, 'There are copers and non-copers and she is one of the non-copers.'

The statement in a measure is true. But what is our

attitude to non-copers? Do we despise them? Does the church despise them?

When Paul talks about the church in 1 Corinthians 12 he describes it as being made up of many parts. Some parts may seem less significant than others, but they are all necessary. In fact, there are no insignificant members of the church. When we take God for our God we take his people for our people. When we claim to be followers of Jesus then we must follow the pattern for living which he set us. That means adopting the same attitude to the weak, the lonely, the outcasts of society, as he did.

Sentiment or love?

How did Jesus approach people? There was nothing sentimental about his approach. So often we confuse real caring with sentimental feelings towards people. I believe that when Jesus approached people he did so with a strong desire to meet them at the very heart of their need. He did not merely come to people to make them happy: indeed, many turned away from Jesus sad (eg the rich young man):

> "Good teacher," he asked, "What must I do to inherit eternal life?"...
>
> Jesus looked at him and loved him. "One thing you lack," he said. "Go, sell everything you have and give to the poor, and you will have treasure in heaven. Then come, follow me."
>
> At this the man's face fell. He went away sad, because he had great wealth (Mk 10:17-22).

Jesus is not opposed to people having wealth, but he knew that this young man's wealth was a barrier to being able fully to commit himself to God. He loved his money more than he loved God, and Jesus loved him too much to fool him into a false sense of security.

Many today seem to feel that as long as we can make people happy then that is enough: a bit like throwing a poor dog a bone every now and then. But Jesus was no sentimentalist. His aim was always to draw people to God, to make them strong in God. He was concerned with their eternal welfare, and sometimes he had to wound in order to heal.

We can think of the Samaritan woman at the well in John 4: Jesus confronted this woman with her past life of sin in order to make her face up to it. He was aware of the woman's discomfort but he pursued the issue in order to help her. Today, many counsellors might want to gloss over the woman's past, to hide it under the carpet and pretend it didn't happen, because they might offend or upset her. But that never helps. Oh, it may give the woman a happy comfortable feeling for a little while, but it would never last. Instead, Jesus gave the woman something far better: he met her at her point of need, which was to make her face up to her past and set her life in order. Love is strong, not weak; it seeks the best for people.

Forgiveness

Love is also accepting. Jesus accepted people as they were. He did not condone sin and always clearly pointed it out, but his love, care and concern shone through. It is all too easy to be quick to judge and point out sin and failure, but if we cannot do it in love we should keep quiet. We need to earn the right to criticise. We need to learn to love people first before we venture into the realm of counselling or confronting.

117

The message which Jesus spoke was clear for all to understand if they listened. He spoke out against sin but cared for the person. The church today is often vague in its message to the world, afraid of giving offence and often confusing love with mere sentiment.

How can and should the church respond to those who have difficulties due to their past experiences or past sin? Our reference point for all that we do, as individual Christians and as the corporate body of the church, must always be the scriptures. So what do they tell us? 'Brothers, if someone is caught in a sin, you who are spiritual should restore him gently' (Gal 6:1). 'Carry each other's burdens, and in this way you will fulfil the law of Christ' (Gal 6:2).

We are encouraged to act, yet how many of us see but do nothing? Evil will prevail when good men do nothing. Jesus commands us to be light in the world to show up the works of darkness. He tells us to be salt to purify and preserve the good in the world. We need to be these things in the world, but how much more do we need to be light and salt in the church?

If we cannot care for people inside the church, dare we attempt to care for those outside? One of the distinguishing features of the early church was their love for one another. But in many churches today we can be so caught up in petty squabbles and in building our own little empires that we become blind to those around us who are in need.

If God offers forgiveness, so should we. If God restores a repentant sinner (just as he has us), so should we be prepared to restore our brothers and sisters and accept them into our fellowships.

Our Lord has many weak children in his family, many dull pupils in his school, many raw soldiers in his army, many

118

lame sheep in his flock. Yet he bears with them all, and casts none away. Happy is that Christian who has learned to do likewise with his brethren.[2]

Offering friendship

Are there any in our church whom we despise because they are not quite in the same social class as us, or are not as intellectual as us, or don't move in the right circles? So often in our places of worship it is the wise, the influential, and those of noble birth who are given prominence, and the poor, the lonely, the unemployed who are neglected. We are taken up by the outward appearance of people while God looks at our hearts.

> Suppose a man comes into your meeting wearing a gold ring and fine clothes, and a poor man in shabby clothes also comes in. If you show special attention to the man wearing fine clothes and say, "Here's a good seat for you," but say to the poor man, "You stand there" or "Sit on the floor by my feet," have you not discriminated among yourselves and become judges with evil thoughts? (Jas 2:2–4)

God instituted the family because he knew that we are sociable beings who need companionship, friendship and human love. The church is God's family—we are his children and he is our Father. In today's society, with an increasing divorce rate and a breakdown of family life, we more than ever need to recapture God's ideal for the church as a family of his people.

The church in a measure usually reflects the social trends of the day. In society today families are more insular, and we have lost the concept of the extended family. We are very concerned to retain our privacy at all costs. It is the individual and the individual's rights which are important. We are less used to mixing with people we don't know well, and we can readily live next door to people for years without knowing anything about them or being interested in them.

Similarly, we can go along to church, sit in our usual place and, instead of becoming part of the wider family of the church, remain in splendid isolation. At the end of the service we may talk to a few select people, but we avoid those that we don't know or don't approve of, or who may want to take up too much of our time. If this happens it is no wonder that many churches are accused of being unfriendly and cliquish and that the stranger, the lonely and the sad go unnoticed.

Difficult people—those with emotional problems, the non-copers—will always gravitate towards the church in the hope of finding help and support. Many of these people are very demanding and can drain the resources of ministers, pastors and others in the church. The knowledge of this tends to make us avoid such time- and energy-consuming people, afraid that if we get involved we will never escape! We often find ourselves exasperated by people who want, as it were, to eat us up because they seem to need so much of us. They want our special and individual attention, and they can stretch us to and beyond our limit of patience, with endless phone calls and demands on our time.

Ministers are all very hard-pressed people with enormous demands being made on them from a variety of sources. I speak as a minister's wife and know that there is always more to do than the minister has time or energy to cope with.

I am not saying, therefore, that we need to make an unqualified response to every person who knocks on our door. That would be very foolish, as we ourselves would soon be worn down and no use to anyone. However, this is where the family of the church can help: there needs to be a sharing of the burden of needy people. In fact we are all needy people, and we all need the help of our fellow brothers and sisters in Christ. But we are all at a different level of need, a level which fluctuates not only from individual to individual but within each of us. There are times when we are able to give comfort and times when we need to receive comfort, times when we are low in emotional and mental resources and other times when we are able to give encouragement.

There should always be this two-way exchange in churches, but so often it becomes a one-way exchange. A few people do all the giving until they are totally exhausted and opt out, and the others, who are many, do all the receiving and taking, often without getting any better.

Those who help others should always have as their aim that the needy person gets better, to the point where he does not need so much human help and is more able to rely directly on God. Likewise, those doing the receiving should be taking active steps to get better, and not merely behave like a sponge, soaking up all the care and attention they can get.

Caring for people in need, no matter what their particular problem, is not an exercise in sentiment. Caring and loving involves being strong for the weaker person—not confirming and sharing their weakness, but endeavouring to help them to be strong. This may involve being firm and even tough with the needy person. Giving in to constant demands and allowing yourself to be manipulated is good neither for you nor for the person you are helping.

There is a time for confronting people just as the

prophet Nathan confronted David over his sin with Bathsheba. There is a time for helping people to acknowledge their past sin, and for encouraging repentance. There is a time to help people see themselves as others see them, a time to exhort them to give up their excuses for their behaviour or to give up their imaginary sick and dependant role. But it must all be done in love. Without love we have no right to speak.

Care and counselling

Unfortunately, many people who get involved in caring and counselling do so to bolster up their own faltering ego. They need to be needed and so they encourage dependence on themselves, which of course is not helpful to either them or their clients.

In recent years there has been an increase in the number of Christian counsellors and counselling services set up. Some of these are helpful and necessary, but there are areas of danger.

Some who set themselves up as 'experts' in this field have little or no formal training. Others consider themselves 'trained counsellors' after attending a conference or series of meetings on counselling, while others may have certificates of bona fide training but are sadly lacking in experience or realism.

The growth in Christian counsellors is in response to Christians who are reluctant to seek help of a psychological nature from anyone other than a Christian. Some of this reluctance may be due to the misconception that it is somehow more respectable to see a Christian counsellor than to see a psychiatrist or psychologist.

It may be further more desirable to go along to a friendly Christian's home where everything is kept quiet and confidential—no one need ever know—than to attend a more public hospital setting.

Obviously where the problem is a spiritual one Christians are right to seek out a wise Christian who can help them. But if their problem is psychological and they refuse to consult a psychiatrist, doctor or counsellor, regardless of whether they are Christian or not, they may delay dealing with their problem until it has reached crisis proportions.

Christians may also set themselves up as counsellors without the proper backing or resources to deal with difficult situations. In this way some Christians may obtain a poorer quality of treatment or even the wrong treatment.

The church is the ideal place, as I believe God intends it to be, for the needy, the lonely and the hurting person to find love. There are those who have experienced rejection in the past, and the people of God can do much to help heal the scars of this by offering acceptance. There are those who have never experienced much of family life or love, and again the church can fill that vacuum. There are single people, a large group for whom the church should fulfil the role of family and friend. The repentant sinner should find forgiveness, not the sound of whispering voices talking about him or her.

As we see more and more of family breakdown in our world, the church has to be in the forefront of caring for those who have experienced such heartbreak. It should also give a clear message to the world about God's love and forgiveness, but also of his intolerance of sin. The family of God can be an example to a needy world of family life where people can come to find healing in their midst.

The church family can be a powerful healing balm. The kind of people that this book is about need acceptance, love and friendship if they are to be free of their past, and the church can give that. For those with mental illness the church family can act as a buffer against the harsh realities of the world in which we live. But we can also have the opposite effect. We too can reject and add to the pain suffered in the past by someone. We can add to the loneliness of the single person by placing undue emphasis on marriage, or add to the pain of the childless by an insensitivity to their personal disappointment. Not everyone falls into the pattern of getting married and having children. Not everyone is able to cope with the stresses of life, not everyone has had a happy childhood; many are living with past memories of painful or sinful incidents which make them difficult to get close to—but what would Christ's response to such people be?

'Come to me all you who are weary and burdened, and I will give you rest' (Mt 11:28).

The church should be Christ's arms to embrace, his feet to go and seek out the lonely and hurting, his eyes and ears to see and hear a world of need.

13

Jesus the Healer of Broken Emotions

Therefore, since we have a great high priest who has gone through the heavens, Jesus the Son of God, let us hold firmly to the faith we profess. For we do not have a high priest who is unable to sympathise with our weaknesses, but we have one who has been tempted in every way, just as we are—yet was without sin. Let us then approach the throne of grace with confidence, so that we may receive mercy and find grace to help us in our time of need (Heb 4:14–16).

We find through life that people often let us down. Even those closest to us can fail to sense our need or fail to respond to it. Even the church may fail. But there is one who will never fail us, who is always ready to listen to us and who understands our deepest needs: Jesus, our High Priest.

Distressed by the pressures of life, haunted by their past and unable to face tomorrow, some people seek oblivion in alcohol or drugs. Others take tranquillisers to help them cope with day-to-day pressures. Some turn to doctors. Others turn to the expert on stress and living with past experiences—the psychiatrist. Is there another means of help for the Christian?

Paul under pressure

The apostle Paul was a man with a past; a past which had the capacity to haunt him and render him useless as God's servant. If Paul had allowed it, his past memories would have constantly told him that he was unfit to teach anyone about Jesus: Paul, the man who had hounded the Christians and who stood by gladly watching Stephen's martyrdom; Paul, the man whose aim had been to crush the early church and who did all in his power to effect that aim.

How did Paul deal with his past? We have a clue in Philippians 3:13–14: 'But one thing I do: Forgetting what is behind and straining towards what is ahead, I press on towards the goal to win the prize for which God has called me heavenwards in Christ Jesus.'

When Paul here talks of forgetting the past I do not think he meant that he erased it from his mind. Indeed, elsewhere Paul describes himself as the chief of sinners. Rather, it was forgetting in the sense of letting it go. There is a world of difference in these two kinds of forgetting. Trying to erase memories from our mind is very difficult and not always helpful. Memories, especially visual and auditory ones, can flash into our minds, time and time again, when we least expect or desire them. These memories can be devastatingly real, and bring with them all the emotions we felt at the time of the event. We need help to forget these images and put them behind us. But there is another kind of forgetting which does not necessarily aim at mind erasure. The old saying 'I'll forgive but I can never forget' is commonly heard. That kind of forgiveness is not true forgiveness because in the remembering of the event the emotions and hurt are remembered too, and bitterness grows as the grudge is borne. That kind of forgiveness is merely empty words. But there is a forgetting which can remember the event but forget the anger, the pain and the sorrow caused by it. This latter kind of remembering of the past does us no harm, whereas the former is destructive.

Putting the past behind us is an act of the will. We determine to leave the past where it belongs.

The apostle Paul did not have a carefree easy life. He was single, so he had no wife to comfort him and share his trials. Like the Lord Jesus he seems not to have had any permanent home of his own. He shares with the Corinthians something of his difficulties: 'For when we came into Macedonia, this body of ours had no rest, but we were harassed at every turn—conflicts on the outside, fears within' (2 Cor 7:5).

Paul was not superhuman, he too experienced conflict and fear. Earlier he says: 'We were under great pressure, far beyond our ability to endure, so that we despaired even of life' (2 Cor 1:8). And again, 'We are hard pressed on every side, but not crushed; perplexed, but not in despair; persecuted, but not abandoned; struck down, but not destroyed' (2 Cor 4:8–9).

God sends help

Paul was not captive to these pressures and problems. They did not limit his service for or communion with God. How did Paul live above the pressures of life? In each of these passages we have looked at he goes on to give the answer: 'But God, who comforts the downcast, comforted us by the coming of Titus' (2 Cor 7:6). God sent Paul and his companions a friend. Human warmth and comfort are important, God knows that. That is why the family within the church is so important. Perhaps God wants us to be a Titus to someone who is downcast: I have certainly known the friendship and comfort of many such Titus figures at times when I have been feeling low, and these dear friends mean much to me. Titus was sent by God to Paul.

At other times God's help was of a different nature:

> But this happened that we might not rely on ourselves but on God, who raises the dead. He has delivered us from such a deadly peril, and he will deliver us. On him we have set our hope that he will continue to deliver us, as you help us by your prayers (2 Cor 1:9–10).

Paul recognises a strength greater than his own. Often when we find ourselves struggling with pressures and stresses, past memories and events, our struggle is due to the fact that we are trying to manage in our own strength. The fact that we, as Christians, have pressures and problems from our past is neither wrong nor odd. It is what we do with those pressures and problems which is important. Do we struggle on in our own strength, or recognise a strength greater than our own, as Paul did? Paul knew his own weaknesses. He knew he needed God. He also knew that he needed other Christians, '...as you help us by your prayers.' Just as he needed Titus' friendship and comfort, he also needed friends to pray for him.

The exchanged life

There is one more answer which Paul found, the greatest help of all:

> We always carry around in our body the death of Jesus, so that the life of Jesus may also be revealed in our body. For

we who are alive are always being given over to death for Jesus' sake, so that his life may be revealed in our mortal body. So then, death is at work in us, but life is at work in you (2 Cor 4:10–11).

Hudson Taylor, the founder of the China Inland Mission, used to talk about 'the exchanged life' and how this enabled him to cope with the many pressures of life. If only we could let this lesson sink deep into our minds and grasp the reality of what Christ in his death has done for us. He not only died to save us from our sins and secure for us eternal life, he died in order to give us his life. He lives in us. When we become Christians we take on Christ in all his fullness.

In evangelical circles we speak of receiving Jesus into our hearts, often to the neglect of the equally dominant truth of our being engrafted into Christ. Indeed, the Greek in John's Gospel can time and time again be translated as 'believing into' Christ, ie, into union with him by faith. Our puny sinful weak lives are engrafted into his pure strong life. We now have a different life source: the exchange is made.

This is quite mind-boggling, and because we find it hard to believe, we live as if it has not happened. It is only when we let this truth dawn on our souls that we will begin to draw from that life-giving sap which Christ has made available to us by his death. When we can reckon ourselves dead to our sin and the damaging effects of our past, and alive in Christ, we will begin on the road to freedom.

It was by dwelling and abiding in the risen Christ that Paul was able to surmount his circumstances, his past failures, hurts and disappointments, and the daily pressures of living. By dependence on God and on the life that Christ exchanged for his own, Paul was able to realise the fruit-bearing potential of his suffering. In this way he allowed his past to have a constructive effect on his life rather than a destructive one.

I would not want to minimise the problems some people have with their past. The scars that the past can inflict are deep and painful. Our past experiences are largely responsible for the type of personality we have. When we become Christians we do not lose our personality, nor are we brainwashed into forgetting our past. So how does this 'exchanged' life work?

Jesus describes himself in John's Gospel as the true vine (Jn 15:1–8). He describes our becoming Christians in terms of being grafted into himself, the true vine. From the moment a branch is grafted into another growing living plant it begins to draw on the sap of that plant. Therefore, from that moment on it has a new life-giving source. However, it may take some considerable time before that life-giving sap changes the ingrafted branch so that it resembles the new parent plant. I know very little about gardening, but I am told by reliable sources that a branch from a cherry or other fruit tree which bears sour fruit can be cut off and grafted into a sweet fruit-bearing tree, and eventually that grafted-in branch from the sour fruit tree will bear sweet fruit, *but it takes time*. The important thing is that it now has a new life-giving sap. This is the same for us, and it is no accident that Jesus chose this analogy. When we become Christians we immediately begin to draw new life from Christ, our new source of life. But it will take time for that new life to transform us into looking like and behaving like Jesus, our new life source.

Overcoming sin

As long as the grafted branch continues to draw on its new life source it will grow and change, but if anything should obstruct the flow it will die, or at best grow slowly and poorly.

So too with us, our transformation into the likeness of Christ is not automatic. We need to draw daily, and minute by minute, on Christ's life. His life and strength are freely available to us but we can affect the rate of flow. Sin will adversely affect the flow of life from him to us. We cannot expect to enjoy God's blessing and help while we entertain sin in our own lives. Perhaps that seems a rather obvious thing to say. But countless Christians are living exactly like that. Sin has to be recognised as sin, for we prefer to dress it up and call it many other things. We say, 'I have a bad temper—it's my personality, I can't help it.' Or a husband may say, 'I like admiring and looking at other women, I just like to appreciate their beauty.' Or a wife may say, 'I complain and moan at my husband and children all day, but they deserve it.'

There are, of course, more serious ways in which we camouflage our sin. A husband may go along to church with his family every Sunday, pretending to be a loving husband and father, while cheating on his wife. We may fill in our tax returns falsely, but deny any wrong in it because we feel that the government shouldn't have so much of our money: they are really cheating us and we are correcting the balance.

We cannot expect victory in our lives while we are living a double or deceitful life. This may be an important reason why so many Christians fail to experience true freedom in Christ from their past. Many of their faults, which they excuse as being 'part of their personality', may more appropriately be called sinfulness.

But by far the main reason for our inability to cope with the past or indeed the present is, I believe, a failure to grasp the truth of the gospel of the indwelling Christ and the power available to us.

Jesus is not only our friend and constant companion, he is the very source of our new life. If we say that our personality, or our past, or our circumstances are too hard for Christ to help us with, then we are failing to recognise who Jesus is. If we say, 'I believe Christ has the power to help but he won't,' then we are again denying the truth of the gospel. The unwillingness is not on Christ's part—but it may be on our part. We may not be willing to give up our past or our weaknesses or our sin.

Compassion and confrontation

Jesus, when he lived on earth, was never afraid to confront his followers or would-be followers. His love was no sentimental desire to see people with a happy smile despite a broken life. He wanted to see those broken lives mended even if it meant initial pain, heartsearching and exposure.

When Jesus met the rich young ruler he knew that the young man's riches were a hindrance to true communion with God. Jesus never settled for half measures. He didn't say to the young man, 'Really you ought to do something about your great wealth, but never mind, follow me as best as you can.' No, Jesus confronted him with the truth of the situation. He didn't fool the young man into a false sense of security. Securing eternal life for us was to cost Jesus dearly: this

132

is not something we can trifle carelessly with. We cannot accept Christ's standards and teachings one day, only to reject them when we are tired or preoccupied with someone or something else. Jesus told the young man the truth, he exposed his need and waited for his response. Sadly the young man walked away, little realising what he was rejecting for the sake of holding on to some worldly wealth, which one day he would have no choice but to leave behind.

When we come to Jesus with our difficulties—either in the past or the present—he will not throw us a sticking-plaster to cover over the hurt. He will come to us with all the tenderness and compassion of one who loved us enough to die for us, but he will also come boldly to show us clearly what we should do. He may confront us with areas of sin in our lives. He may be firm in telling us to forget the past and press on to what is ahead. He may command us to forgive as we have been forgiven. We can either listen and obey, or be like the rich ruler and turn sadly away.

One thing is sure: we have a Saviour who is not untouched by our heartaches, our difficulties, our sore circumstances or our failures. He has suffered more than we ever will. A man with a past, yes. He was born with the stigma of illegitimacy hanging over him (in those days this was a serious social disgrace). He was born of poor parents, who didn't even have a proper cradle for him or baby clothes when he was born. He was misunderstood by friends and relatives. He was spurned by the religious leaders of his day. He had no home to call his own, no wife or children to comfort him. He was let down by those he loved. He was abandoned by his closest friends and betrayed by one of them. Ultimately he suffered a humiliating public trial and execution after being falsely accused. And after all that, he suffered intense loneliness as he felt abandoned by God. Have we suffered more?

Who could be a better psychotherapist, friend and counsellor than Jesus? Although Jesus may choose to work through human agencies, ultimately it is in him that we find the healer of broken emotions.

14

God in Every Circumstance

> I had not learned to think of God as the one great Circumstance in whom we live and move and have our being, and of all lesser circumstances as necessarily the kindest, wisest, best, because either ordered or permitted by Him. Hence my disappointment and trial were very great (James Hudson Taylor).[1]

As Hudson Taylor experienced, so do we. When we do not recognise God as the 'circumstance' in which we move and have our being, our disappointments may be very great indeed.

God's plan—or ours?

When my husband, Harry, and I were married we planned our life together. This plan included a life-long career as missionaries and about six children. The first part of our plan went wrong when we were obliged, after a little less than two years, to leave our missionary posts in Iran owing to the revolution there. Our disappointment was great. We had planned to spend, apart from furloughs, the rest of our lives there.

Not put off altogether, we went out to Pakistan to resume our missionary career. After only a few weeks I became ill. My illness lasted several months and after only seven months in Pakistan I was advised to return home for medical tests and treatment. The memory of our unplanned departure from Iran came rushing into our minds and our immediate thought was, 'Not again.' We planned that I would return home on my own for a spell to regain my health, and then return to Pakistan. However, again *our* plan was to be thwarted. Medical advice was against my return. It was considered that my physical constitution could not withstand the health hazards of life in Pakistan. Harry was obliged to pack up and return home to me in Scotland. It was to take me three years fully to regain my health, during which time many friends wrote me off as a physical and psychological wreck. Again, our disappointment was great.

The next part of our plan to go wrong concerned children. We discovered that not only were we not to have six children, we were unable to have any natural children of our own. I have already written a book about that experience so suffice it to say here that this was a great sadness.

There have been other disappointments along the way. For me one of the greatest was being misunderstood by friends. When we returned home from Iran there were family and friends who said we should have come home sooner. We had waited on to see how the situation would develop after Khomeini's return—in fact we were flown out by the RAF along with other missionaries and expatriates. Other friends thought we had thrown in the towel too soon!

A similar situation arose when we returned from Pakistan. Many of our friends found it hard to understand that God could take us out to the missionary field again for such a short period of time. It was easier for them to assume that we had got our guidance wrong, and should never have gone abroad in the first place.

It is difficult enough to cope with your own personal disappointments, without having to cope with well-meaning but misguided friends as well, but such is life and these are part of the circumstances we often find ourselves in.

Now, as Harry and I look back over the past thirteen years since we made *our* plans, we are able to see something of *God's* plan for our lives. There is a beautiful story which Amy Carmichael tells in one of her books. It is about an embroidery cloth; on one side it looks a mess, with bits of thread going all over the place. On the other side is the beautiful picture which is being embroidered. Our lives are a bit like that. Often we see only the reverse side, which looks a bit of a mess at times, and we can't understand or see where all the threads are going to. But God looks from above and sees the beautiful picture which the strands of cotton are making.

At times we felt that our lives looked in a bit of a mess. We knew a sense of failure and perplexity. We couldn't understand why God should lead us along such a strange path. Yet we were able to hold on to the knowledge that God had been leading us. Through the mist we were able to see God's hand, and that brought comfort and peace which cushioned our natural disappointment. The Master tapestry-maker was controlling the threads of circumstance in our lives and we had no need to fear.

Shaping our lives

There is a hymn written by William Cowper (a man who knew much darkness in his life) which speaks of God's providence. I will quote only two verses.[2]

> Ye fearful saints, fresh courage take;
> The clouds ye so much dread
> Are big with mercy, and shall break
> In blessings on your head.
>
> Judge not the Lord by feeble sense,
> But trust him for his grace;
> Behind a frowning providence
> He hides a smiling face.

Now as we are able to see something of the wonder of God's plan for our lives, we are more than a little convinced that his plan has been best. My husband is now very happy as a minister in the Church of Scotland, and his ministry is greatly enhanced because of our experiences abroad. We now have three beautiful adopted children, and when I look at these little ones I realise that had we been able to have our own children we would never have had these adopted ones, and our lives would have been the poorer for it.

We cannot say as Christians that any of our experiences, excepting deliberate sin, are redundant, although God is big enough to capitalise even on our sin. Some of life's sorest experiences bring some of our richest joys. I remember when we were in Iran and feeling quite useless as we tried to master the language, able to communicate only at the level of a three-year-old, Harry and I discussed our purpose in Iran. It seemed even then, before we realised how short our stay there was to be, that God had already indicated to us that our time there was not so much so that we could benefit anyone else, but rather that God was at work in our own lives. We learned a lesson there which we have never forgotten. God is more interested in *who we are* and what we become than in *what we do*. We tend to be service-centred, whereas God is person-centred. We can get so involved in Christian service that we neglect our own personal walk with God. Circumstances are God's tool to shape and mould our lives.

So often we are anxious for God to change our circumstances while what God wants is change in us.

God uses our pain

What about our circumstances and experiences before we became Christians? What of those who have suffered physical or sexual abuse as children, what of those who have been raped or had other similar horrifying experiences? Are these events part of God's plan for our lives? These are difficult questions, but we believe that while God is not the author of sin or evil, he does permit it. The cross is an example of this. Christ's crucifixion and death were part of God's plan for Jesus, but he was not the author of the evil in the hearts of the men who carried out the crucifixion. Rather, God permitted and used their evil to execute his own plan.

It may seem a harsh thing to say, but if we believe that God chose us to be his own even before creation, as Paul tells us in Ephesians 1:4, then we have to believe that our pre-Christian lives are as much God's plan for us as our post-conversion lives, and that must include the bad experiences as well as the good ones.

Theologians make a distinction between what God

decrees and what God permits. I'm not saying that God decreed the evil which may have surrounded our early lives, but he has permitted it and intends to use it constructively in our lives if we will allow him.

How could sexual abuse be part of God's plan? I do not claim to know all the answers, for some things will remain a mystery until we see the full picture of the tapestry when we reach heaven. However, there are many people who have suffered in terrible ways, both before and after they have become Christians, who have been able to see part of God's plan in allowing their suffering.

Paul indicates something of the purpose:

> Praise be to the God and Father of our Lord Jesus Christ, the Father of compassion and the God of all comfort, who comforts us in all our troubles, so that we can comfort those in any trouble with the comfort we ourselves have received from God (2 Cor 1:3–4).

There was a time when I wondered why God had allowed me the pain of two miscarriages and ultimate childlessness. Yet now I can look back and see how he has enabled me to comfort and help others in a similar position. In the same way, things which happened way back in my childhood have helped to make me a stronger person. It's a bit like the struggle of the butterfly to escape his cocoon—it makes him the stronger.

If we have never had to grapple with painful events in our lives, if we have known nothing but a life of ease, then I would suspect that we are of little use in helping others.

We live in a real world, not a make-believe fairy tale. We live with all the horrors of pain, violence and evil. Some of our past painful experiences may equip us to cope better with our adult life, as well as enabling us to help others.

All these events in our lives present us with choices. We can choose to allow them to envelop us, chaining us to a memory which limits our service for God and our joy in him. Or we can see these events as stepping stones to discovering new dimensions in God's love, compassion, power and grace.

Because of its obvious relevance I would like to finish this chapter by quoting a favourite hymn of mine by Frederick William Faber (1814-63).

> Workman of God! O lose not heart,
> But learn what God is like,
> And, in the darkest battlefield,
> Thou shalt know where to strike.
>
> Thrice blest is he to whom is given
> The instinct that can tell
> That God is on the field when he
> Is most Invisible.
>
> He hides himself so wondrously,
> As though there were no God;
> He is least seen when all the powers
> Of ill are most abroad.
>
> Ah! God is other than we think;
> His ways are far above,
> Far beyond reason's height, and reached
> Only by childlike love.
>
> Then learn to scorn the praise of men,
> And learn to lose with God;
> For Jesus won the world through Shame,
> And beckons thee his road.

For right is right, since God is God,
And right the day must win;
To doubt would be disloyalty,
To falter would be sin.

15

A Foretaste of Heaven

I am not so naive as to think that I have all the answers, or even a good number of them, to the problems we face in dealing with our past hurts, disappointments and sin. But I hope that we have begun to look at some of the issues involved and shed a little light into the dark tunnel which our past can create for us.

It would be foolish to suggest that we can know complete freedom in every realm of our past experiences. What we aim for, though, depends on our relationship with our heavenly Father. Do we believe he cares? Do we believe he knows our agonies? Do we believe his grace is sufficient as Paul reminds us? 'My grace is sufficient for you, for my power is made perfect in weakness' (2 Cor 12:9).

'All kinds of trials'

We cannot attain perfection in this life; we are chasing rainbows if we think we can. We will have to wait until we reach heaven, or Jesus returns, before we can know perfect freedom from our fallen natures and the effects on us of a fallen world. What we have been promised is a foretaste of heaven here on earth. Jesus promises us peace, inner peace which is not disturbed by our circumstances. But even the quality of our peace and joy are poor in contrast to what we shall experience in glory. Because of our fallen nature, our ability to appropriate for ourselves all that Christ has made available for us is restricted. Think of a light connection which has partly corroded. The power for the light is there and sufficient. The light bulb is also there, waiting to be connected to the power source. But the light shines bright at times and dim at other times because of the corrosion at the point of contact. We cannot escape the reality of the existence of sin and evil in our world. The devil is alive and well and working hard to put as much corrosion at our connecting point as possible.

Talking about family life in her book *What is a Family?* Edith Schaeffer says something which is equally applicable to our subject:

> The trouble is that people want *more* than the Lord promises; they want the state of perfection that will not come until Jesus comes back to change us. Wanting more than we can have now, we have another case of "everything or nothing", and so many times it ends up "nothing".[1]

What are we promised?

In his great mercy he has given us new birth into a living hope through the resurrection of Jesus Christ from the dead, and into an inheritance that can never perish, spoil or fade—kept in heaven for you, who through faith are shielded by God's power until the coming of salvation that is ready to be revealed in the last time. In this you greatly rejoice, though now for a little while you may have had to suffer grief in all kinds of trials. These have come so that your faith—of greater worth than gold, which perishes even though refined by fire—may be proved genuine and may result in praise, glory and honour when Jesus Christ is revealed (1 Pet 1:3–7).

These words, and many more like them in the Bible, are written to encourage us. This life is not all we have; we have a glorious hope and future. But does this mean that we just give up on this present life and look to our future in eternity? No. That would be like the Romans who asked Paul if they should keep on sinning so that grace might increase, because where there is more sin there is more grace.

Paul tells us in his letter to the Corinthians about his 'thorn in the flesh'. He doesn't tell us exactly what it was, and that is good, because the actual thorn is irrelevant. The point is that here was something in Paul's life which he did not like. It caused him a great deal of pain and discomfort, perhaps even embarrassment. He not only asked God to remove it, he pleaded with God three times. But God said 'No'. God's answer was not cruel and unfeeling, but he knew what was best for Paul.

Did this thorn in the flesh disqualify Paul from serving God? No, indeed, Paul saw this as part of God's equipment for service.

> To keep me from becoming conceited because of these surpassingly great revelations, there was given me a thorn in my flesh, a messenger of Satan, to torment me. Three times I pleaded with the Lord to take it away from me. But he said to me, "My grace is sufficient for you, for my power is made perfect in weakness" (2 Cor 12:7–9).

What was Paul's reaction to this thorn in the flesh and to God's refusal to take it away? Was he bitter and angry? Did he decide to opt out of serving God because of it?

Therefore I will boast all the more gladly about my weaknesses, so that Christ's power may rest on me. That is why, for Christ's sake, I delight in weaknesses, in insults, in hardships, in persecutions, in difficulties. For when I am weak, then I am strong (2 Cor 12:9–10).

In our prayers to be free of our past, we need to leave room for the possibility that our very past may be part of God's equipment for us to serve him better. We do not use our past as an excuse for our lack of joy in Christ, but rather the cause of greater joy.

Into the future

No matter what our difficulty or past experience is, God is a God of new beginnings. He gave Jonah a fresh start after his disobedience in refusing to go to Nineveh. He gave Elijah a new start after his bout of depression in the wilderness. He gave Peter a new beginning and a new commission to service after his failure.

God can capitalise on our past and use it to help us in the future. God can equally heal our broken lives, torn apart and shattered by man's inhumanity to man. No past, no personality, no act of sin or disobedience is too bad or difficult for him. His grace is sufficient.

Memories, good or bad, need to be seen through the spectacles of scriptural teaching. The bad memories we lay at Christ's feet asking for his grace to leave them in the past, taking into the present and future only the lessons from them which he can use to equip us better for service. The good memories we come and thank Jesus for. We cherish them and allow them to be a spur to greater faith in God.

God frequently encouraged the Israelites to remember their past suffering in Egypt and to remember how

God delivered them. In fact, a special annual feast day was appointed so that the children of Israel for generations to come would remember the slavery in and deliverance from Egypt:

> Observe the month of Abib and celebrate the Passover of the Lord your God, because in the month of Abib he brought you out of Egypt by night...so that all the days of your life you may remember the time of your departure from Egypt (Deut 16:1–3).

Some of the memories for the children of Israel must have been painful, but these were contrasted with God's mighty deliverance.

As Christians we celebrate another Passover. Jesus was God's Passover lamb to bring us a greater deliverance than the children of Israel had. Theirs was but a foreshadowing of what was to come, but we have the reality of Christ's redeeming work in our hearts.

Can we contrast any past hurts, failure or sin with the deliverance which God has provided for us through Jesus?

The world offers escapism which, either through drink or drugs or some other method, offers oblivion— or at least the possibility of obscuring the past for us. We can for a while pretend it didn't happen. But the freedom from the past which God offers us is escape— true deliverance. When by God's help we are delivered from, or escape from our past, he enables us to face the reality of it without reliving the horror or being destroyed by it.

We live in a world which exalts man; in secular thought, man is the centre of the universe. As Christians we must resist this kind of thinking, for God is the centre of our world.

It is easy, and sometimes pleasant, to talk for hours

about all our problems, about past experiences, traumas and difficulties. It is much harder to get on with the business of working through these difficulties with a view to overcoming them. But if we have God in the centre of our lives, he will give us motivation and strength, and we will be amazed to see how much fruit our hard work will bear.

We are called to be free, and that includes freedom from the binding chains of the past.

Brothers, I do not consider myself yet to have taken hold of it. But one thing I do: Forgetting what is behind and straining toward what is ahead, I press on towards the goal to win the prize for which God has called me heavenwards in Christ Jesus (Phil 3:13–14).

Notes

Chapter 1

1. Thomas Watson, *The Lord's Prayer* (Banner of Truth Trust: Edinburgh, 1979), p 3.
2. C S Lewis, *The Last Battle* (Fontana Lions: London, 1980), pp 135–140.

Chapter 2

1. Richard Foster, *Celebration of Discipline* (Hodder & Stoughton: London, 1981), p 4.

Chapter 3

1. Ian H Murray, *D Martyn Lloyd Jones, The First Forty Years, 1899–1939* (Banner of Truth Trust: Edinburgh, 1982), opposite p 1.
2. C S Lewis, *The Screwtape Letters* (Fontana: Glasgow, 1976), p 17.
3. A W Tozer, *Leaning into the Wind* (Kingsway: Eastbourne, 1985), p 34.

Chapter 9

1. C R Vaughan, *The Gifts of the Holy Spirit* (Banner of Truth Trust: Edinburgh, 1975), p 213.
2. J C Ryle, *Holiness* (Evangelical Press: Bridgend, Centenary Edition 1879–1979), p 29.
3. John White, *The Fight* (IVP: Leicester, 1977), p 114.
4. J C Ryle, *op cit* p 88.
5. J C Ryle, *op cit* p 92.

Chapter 10

1. Thomas Watson, *The Lord's Prayer* (Banner of Truth Trust: Edinburgh, 1979), p 3.

Chapter 11

1. J A C Brown, *Freud and the Post-Freudians* (Penguin: Harmondsworth, 1961), p 117.
2. *ibid* p 43.
3. Charles Rycroft, *A Critical Dictionary of Psychoanalysis* (Penguin: Harmondsworth, 1972), p xvii.

Chapter 12

1. J C Ryle, *Holiness* (Evangelical Press: Bridgend, Centenary Edition 1879–1979), p 213.
2. John Blanchard, *More Gathered Gold* (Evangelical Press: Bridgend, 1986), p 47.

Chapter 14

1. Dr and Mrs Howard Taylor, *Biography of James Hudson Taylor* (China Inland Overseas Missionary Fellowship, 1965), p 119.
2. William Cowper, God moves in a mysterious way.

Chapter 15

1. Edith Schaeffer, *What is a Family?* (Hodder & Stoughton: London, 1976), p 213.

Emotionally Free

by Rita Bennett

'One of the great words in the Bible is freedom. God wants you to be yourself, not what someone else wanted or wants you to be. Not bound in your emotions and memories, but free—free to live now and free to look ahead with confidence.'

'He wants you to find out who you are, and to enjoy being you. He wants you to be free to love Him with all your being, just as He loves you. Free to love yourself, your family and your neighbours. Free to cry, to laugh, to love.'

This book will show you how to let Jesus heal the inner hurts that would steal your joy and peace. It tells of real people with real problems—and how they found answers—so that you too can enjoy the freedom God intends for all His people.

RITA BENNETT is also author of *How to Pray for Inner Healing* and *Making Peace with Your Inner Child*, and co-author with her husband Dennis of *The Holy Spirit and You* and *Trinity of Man*.

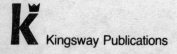

Kingsway Publications

Making Peace with Your Inner Child

by Rita Bennett

In a world that longs for peace, Christians have the promise of peace from God. Sadly, however, many believers have lived with inner turmoil since their childhood. In *Making Peace with Your Inner Child* Rita Bennett gives practical insights on how to receive emotional healing. She pays particular attention to childhood memories, showing how we can receive healing from hurts inflicted even long ago.

Throughout the book there are examples and prayers that will minister to all those who suffer from emotional trauma.

Rita Bennett is Vice-President of the Christian Renewal Association in Washington. This is the third volume in her series on inner healing, following on from *Emotionally Free* and *How to Pray for Inner Healing*.

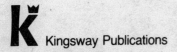

Kingsway Publications

A Child—At Any Cost?

by Mary Mealyea

'Have you heard Irene's news? She's expecting in April. She always wanted a Spring baby. Isn't it wonderful!'

The birth of a child—a cause for great rejoicing. Yet that very joy can wound the heart of those who are denied the precious gift of parenthood.

Mary Mealyea longed to be a mother, just like her friends. But she came to see that genuine understanding was scarce, and honest talk nearly impossible. More than that, she faced a long series of medical hurdles, fraught with ethical decisions and challenges that would put a strain on her relationship with her husband. And with her God.

Mary (known to her friends as 'Ray') shares her story to allow others to understand the trauma of infertility. In addition, her own medical training will help those who are walking the same path to evaluate current options in treatment. Most of all, we see how pain and affliction can come to enrich a Christian's walk with her Lord.

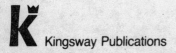

Kingsway Publications